DASH DIET

COOKBOOK

for Beginners

1900 DAYS OF HEALTHY, LOW-SODIUM, HIGH-POTASSIUM RECIPES THAT TASTE DELICIOUS.

By

Diana Martinez

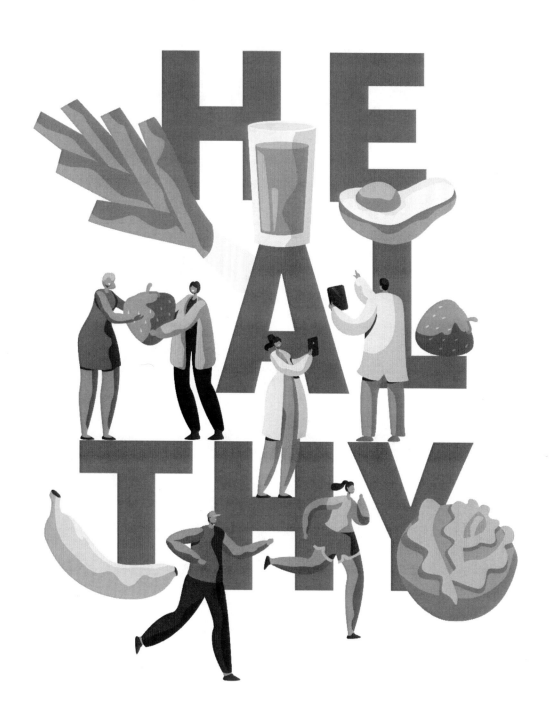

Table of content

Introduction

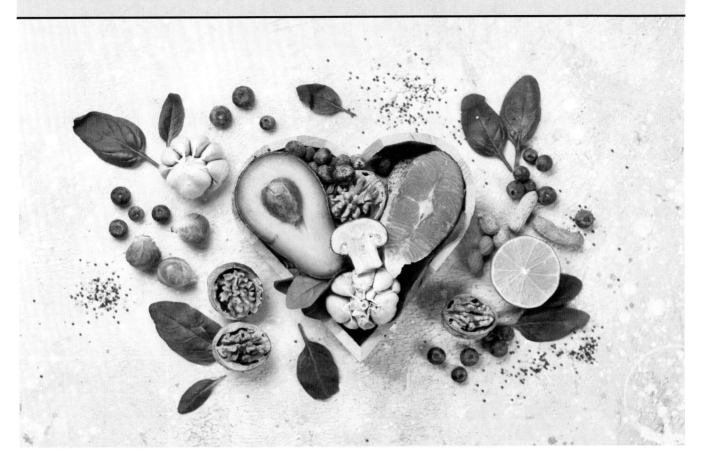

Welcome to the world of the DASH diet! If you're reading this, chances are you're interested in improving your health, eating more nutrient-dense foods, and living your best life. And let me tell you, you're in the right place.

The DASH diet has been around for a few decades, but it's only recently started gaining mainstream popularity. And for a good reason: this eating plan is not only delicious, but it's also incredibly healthy.

It's been proven to lower blood pressure, reduce the risk of heart disease and stroke, and improve overall health and well-being.

So, what is the DASH diet, exactly? Well, it stands for Dietary Approaches to Stop Hypertension. It was initially developed by the National Heart, Lung, and Blood Institute (NHLBI) to help lower blood pressure without medication. The diet emphasizes whole, nutrient-dense foods and limits processed and high-sodium foods.

The fundamental principles of the DASH diet are straightforward: eat a variety of whole, nutrient-dense foods and products; limit intake of processed foods, saturated fats, and added sugars; reduce sodium intake by choosing low-sodium options and avoiding high-sodium foods; and balance calorie intake with physical activity to achieve and maintain a healthy weight.

But here's the thing: the DASH diet is not a one-size-fits-all approach, and it's not about counting calories or cutting out entire food groups. Instead, it's about making healthy choices and building a balanced diet that works for you.

That's where this book comes in. Over 200 delicious, healthy recipes per the DASH diet principles. But these recipes aren't just good for you but also delicious. We've got you covered from breakfast to dinner, snacks to desserts.

So, how did we come up with these recipes? Well, it was challenging, and I wanted to ensure that each recipe was healthy but also flavorful and satisfying. So, I tested and re-tested each recipe until I was sure it was perfect. I made sure to include a wide variety of dishes so that there's something for everyone.

But here's the thing: the DASH diet is not about deprivation. It's not about cutting out all your favorite foods and subsisting on bland salads and steamed vegetables. Instead, it's about finding a balance between healthy choices and indulgences. That's why you'll find plenty of delicious, comforting dishes in this book – from lasagna to stir-fry, mac and cheese to chocolate cake.

Of course, I ensured that each recipe aligned with the DASH diet principles. That means using plenty of fruits and vegetables, choosing lean proteins like chicken and fish, opting for whole grains like brown rice and quinoa, and using minimal added sugars and saturated fats. I also ensured to keep sodium levels in check by using plenty of herbs and spices for flavor rather than relying on salt.

But here's the thing: the DASH diet is not just about your food. It's also about the way you eat. That means enjoying your meals, savoring each bite, and being mindful of your hunger and fullness cues. It means cooking at home more often and planning your meals and snacks. And it means being active and getting plenty of exercise, whether going for a walk, hitting the gym, or trying out.

If you're looking for a healthy eating plan backed by science to help you achieve your health goals, the DASH diet is a great place to start. Not only is it delicious and satisfying, but it's also been shown to offer several health benefits that can help you live your best life.

One of the key benefits of the DASH diet is its ability to lower blood pressure. High blood pressure, or hypertension, is a common health problem that can increase the risk of heart disease, stroke, and other severe health conditions. The DASH diet has been proven to be an effective way to lower blood pressure, both in people with hypertension and normal blood pressure.

Studies have shown that the DASH diet can lower systolic blood pressure (the top number) by 11 points and diastolic blood pressure (the bottom number) by 6 points in people with hypertension. And even in people with normal blood pressure, the DASH diet can help prevent hypertension from developing in the first place.

But the benefits of the DASH diet continue beyond there. The diet has also been shown to reduce the risk of heart disease and stroke, two leading causes of death worldwide. In addition, by emphasizing whole, nutrient-dense foods and limiting processed and high-sodium foods, the DASH diet helps to lower cholesterol levels and improve overall heart health.

One study found that following the DASH diet for just eight weeks led to significant improvements in several markers of heart health, including LDL ("bad") cholesterol, triglycerides, and blood pressure. And other studies have shown that the DASH diet can reduce the risk of heart disease by as much as 18%, making it one of the most effective dietary approaches for heart health.

But the benefits of the DASH diet go beyond just heart health. The diet has also been shown to help with weight management, diabetes prevention and management, and overall well-being. By focusing on whole, nutrient-dense foods and limiting processed and high-sugar foods, the DASH diet can help you maintain a healthy weight and reduce the risk of type 2 diabetes.

One study found that following the DASH diet was more effective than a low-fat or low-carb diet for reducing insulin resistance, a critical factor in developing type 2 diabetes. And other studies have shown that the DASH diet can improve overall well-being, including reducing the risk of depression, improving cognitive function, and reducing inflammation.

So, how exactly does the DASH diet offer all these health benefits? Well, it's all about the food you eat. The DASH diet emphasizes whole, nutrient-dense foods like fruits, vegetables, whole grains, lean proteins, and low-fat dairy products. These foods are rich in vitamins, minerals, and other essential nutrients for good health.

By contrast, the DASH diet limits processed and high-sodium foods, which can contribute to high blood pressure, heart disease, and other health problems. In addition, processed foods are often high in added sugars, saturated fats, and refined carbohydrates, all of which can lead to inflammation, insulin resistance, and other health issues.

So, by choosing whole, nutrient-dense foods and limiting processed and high-sodium foods, the DASH diet helps to promote overall health and well-being. And the great thing is it's a simple diet to follow. So, with some planning and preparation, anyone can enjoy the delicious, satisfying meals the DASH diet offers.

Whether you want to lower your blood pressure, improve your heart health, or feel your best, the DASH diet is a great way to achieve your health goals.

One way to do this is to start small and gradually change over time. For example, add more fruits and vegetables to your meals or swap processed snacks for whole-grain options. Then, as you get more comfortable with these changes, you can gradually incorporate more DASH-friendly foods into your diet.

Another critical aspect of the DASH diet is the way you eat. The diet emphasizes mindful eating, which means paying attention to your hunger and fullness cues and savoring each bite. This can help you avoid overeating and promote a healthier relationship with food.

In addition to making healthy food choices, staying active and getting plenty of exercises is essential. The DASH diet emphasizes the importance of physical activity and recommends at least 150 minutes of moderate-intensity exercise per week.

This can include activities like walking, jogging, cycling, or swimming and strength-training exercises like weightlifting or bodyweight. By staying active and getting plenty of exercises, you can help maintain a healthy weight, reduce your risk of chronic diseases, and improve your overall health and well-being.

The DASH diet is a delicious, healthy, and sustainable way to achieve your health goals. The DASH diet can help lower blood pressure, improve heart health, promote weight management, and enhance overall well-being by emphasizing whole, nutrient-dense foods and limiting processed and high-sodium foods.

But let's start.

What is the Dash diet?

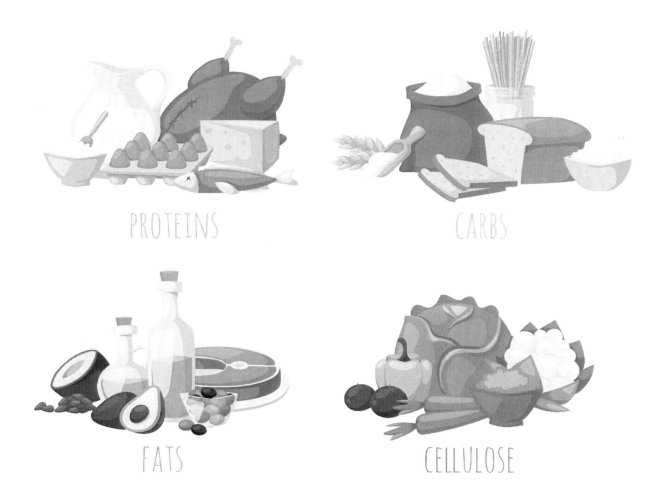

PROTEINS

CARBS

FATS

CELLULOSE

The DASH diet stands for Dietary Approaches to Stop Hypertension. It was initially developed by the National Heart, Lung, and Blood Institute (NHLBI) to help lower blood pressure without medication. But over the years, it's become clear that the DASH diet offers many health benefits, from improving heart health to promoting weight loss.

So, how does the DASH diet work? Well, it's all about choosing the right foods. The DASH diet emphasizes whole, nutrient-dense foods like vegetable, fruits, whole grains, lean proteins, and low-fat dairy products. These foods contain vitamins, minerals, and other essential nutrients for good health.

By contrast, the DASH diet limits processed and high-sodium foods, which can contribute to high blood pressure, heart disease, and other health problems. In addition, processed foods are often high in saturated fats , added sugars, and refined carbohydrates, all of which can lead to inflammation, insulin resistance, and other health issues.

But the DASH diet isn't just about what you eat – it's also about how you eat. The diet emphasizes mindful eating, which means paying attention to your hunger and fullness cues and savoring each bite. This can help you avoid overeating and promote a healthier relationship with food.

So, how do you get started with the DASH diet? Well, here are some simple steps you can take:

Focus on fruits and vegetables. Aim to include at least five servings of fruits and vegetables in your diet each day. Choose a variety of colorful produce, including berries, leafy greens, citrus fruits, and cruciferous vegetables like broccoli and cauliflower.

Choose whole grains. Opt for whole-grain bread, pasta, and cereal instead of refined grains like white bread and rice. Entire grains are richer in nutrients and can help you feel fuller for longer.

Include lean proteins. Choose lean proteins like fish, chicken, beans, and legumes, and limit your intake of red meat and processed meats like bacon and sausage.

Cut back on sodium. Limit sodium intake and do not exceed the threshold of 2,300 milligrams per day (or 1,500 milligrams (or 1,500 milligrams if you have high blood pressure). This means avoiding high-sodium foods like processed snacks, canned soups, and fast food.

Emphasize healthy fats. Choose healthy fats like avocado, olive oil, nuts, and seeds, and limit your intake of saturated and trans fats.

Be mindful of portion sizes. Pay attention to your hunger and fullness cues, and try to eat slowly and mindfully. This can help you avoid overeating and promote a healthier relationship with food.

Get active. The DASH diet emphasizes the importance of physical activity, so try to get at least 150 minutes of moderate-intensity exercise per week. This can include activities like walking, cycling, jogging, or swimming and strength-training exercises like weightlifting or bodyweight.

By following these simple steps, you can start incorporating the principles of the DASH diet into your daily life. And the great thing is it's not a complicated diet. With a bit of planning and preparation, anyone can enjoy the delicious, satisfying meals the DASH diet offers.

So, let's see what the main benefits are of the diet.

Lower blood pressure: The DASH diet has been shown to lower blood pressure in people with hypertension and normal blood pressure. By focusing on whole, nutrient-dense foods and limiting processed and high-sodium foods, the DASH diet can help you maintain healthy blood pressure levels.

Improve heart health: The DASH diet is rich in nutrients like fiber, potassium, and magnesium, which have been shown to improve heart health. In addition, by choosing whole, nutrient-dense foods and limiting saturated and trans fats, the DASH diet edcan help reduce the risk of heart disease and stroke.

Promote weight loss: By emphasizing whole, nutrient-dense foods and limiting processed and high-sugar foods, the DASH diet can help you maintain a healthy weight. And because the diet is rich in fiber and protein, it can help you feel fuller for longer and reduce your overall calorie intake.

Reduce the risk of diabetes: The DASH diet has been shown to reduce the risk of type 2 diabetes by improving insulin resistance. In addition, by choosing whole, nutrient-dense foods and limiting refined carbohydrates and added sugars, the DASH diet can help regulate blood sugar levels and prevent diabetes.

Enhance overall well-being: The DASH diet is rich in nutrients and antioxidants that can help boost overall well-being. In addition, the DASH diet can help reduce inflammation, improve cognitive function, and promote a healthier, happier lifestyle by choosing whole, nutrient-dense foods and limiting processed and high-sugar foods.

But the benefits of the DASH diet aren't just physical – they're also mental and emotional. By emphasizing mindful eating, the DASH diet can help promote a healthier relationship with food and reduce stress and anxiety around eating. And by promoting a healthier, happier lifestyle overall, the DASH diet can help you feel more energized, confident, and fulfilled.

Who Should Follow This Diet

The DASH diet is healthy and can benefit many people, including those with high blood pressure, heart disease, and diabetes, and those looking to maintain a healthy weight or improve their overall health and well-being.

In particular, the DASH diet is often recommended for people with hypertension or high blood pressure. The diet emphasizes whole, nutrient-dense foods and limits processed and high-sodium foods, which can help lower blood pressure.

But even if you don't have high blood pressure, the DASH diet can still be a great way to improve your well-being. Choosing whole, nutrient-dense foods and limiting processed and high-sugar foods can reduce the risk of chronic diseases like heart disease and diabetes and promote weight loss and overall well-being.

Best Diet?

Determining if the DASH diet is proper depends on your health goals, dietary preferences, and medical history. For example, suppose you have a history of hypertension, heart disease, or diabetes, want to maintain a healthy weight, or improve your well-being. In that case, the DASH diet may be an excellent option.

However, talking to your healthcare provider before starting any new dietary or exercise plan is essential, especially if you have underlying medical conditions or take medications. Your health care provider can help you determine whether the DASH diet is appropriate for your needs and provide guidance on safely and effectively incorporating it into your lifestyle.

It's also important to note that the DASH diet is not a one-size-fits-all approach. While the diet emphasizes whole, nutrient-dense foods and limits processed and high-sodium foods, personalizing the diet is still important to meet your individual needs and preferences. For example, suppose you have dietary restrictions or food allergies. In that case, you may need to modify certain aspects of the diet to ensure it meets your nutritional needs.

The DASH diet is a healthy and sustainable eating plan that can benefit many people. But before starting the diet, it's essential to talk to your health care provider to determine if it's the right choice for you and to get personalized guidance on how to make the diet work for your individual needs and goals.

Does It Work

The DASH diet is effective in improving health outcomes for many people. For example, numerous studies have found that the DASH diet can lower blood pressure, improve heart health, promote weight loss, and reduce the risk of chronic diseases like diabetes and cancer.

For example, a large-scale study published in the New England Journal of Medicine found that the DASH diet was more effective than a typical American diet in reducing blood pressure. Other studies have found that the DASH diet can help improve cholesterol levels, reduce inflammation, and improve insulin resistance.

But it's important to note that the effectiveness of the DASH diet depends on various factors, including adherence to the diet, individual health factors, and other lifestyle factors like exercise and stress management. Additionally, the DASH diet is not a quick fix or fad diet: it is a sustainable approach to healthy eating that requires a long-term commitment to making healthy food choices and lifestyle changes. Therefore, although the DASH diet effectively improves health outcomes for many people, it is essential to approach it as a lifestyle change, not as a temporary solution.

By making gradual changes over time and prioritizing whole, nutrient-dense foods, you can reap the DASH diet's many health benefits and achieve long well-being.

How Does the Dash Eating Plan Work

The DASH eating plan emphasizes whole, nutrient-dense foods and limits processed and high-sodium foods. This approach is designed to help lower blood pressure, improve heart health, promote weight loss, and reduce the risk of chronic diseases like diabetes and cancer.

The DASH eating plan emphasizes fruits, vegetables, whole grains, lean proteins, and low-fat dairy products. These foods are rich in nutrients like fibre, vitamins, and minerals. They help provide the body with the energy it needs to function correctly.

By contrast, the DASH eating plan limits processed and high-sodium foods, often high in calories, unhealthy fats, and added sugars. These foods can contribute to weight gain, inflammation, insulin resistance, and other health problems. The DASH eating plan also emphasizes mindful eating, which means paying attention to your hunger and fullness cues and savoring each bite. This can help you avoid overeating and promote a healthier relationship with food.

Additionally, the DASH eating plan recommends limiting alcohol consumption and staying active with regular exercise. These lifestyle factors can further improve health outcomes and well-being overall well-being.

The DASH eating plan gives the body the nutrients to function correctly while limiting unhealthy foods that contribute to chronic diseases and other health problems. You can achieve benight and well-being by prioritizing whole, nutrient-dense foods and adopting a healthy, active lifestyle.

Tips For Dash Diet Success

The DASH diet can be a powerful tool for improving well-being and well-being. Still, success with the diet requires commitment and effort. However, by following a few essential tips, you will achieve your set goals and improve your health. These tips include starting with minor changes, planning, emphasizing whole, nutrient-dense foods, limiting processed and high-sodium foods, being mindful of portion sizes, staying hydrated, and staying active. By taking care of these tips daily, you can create an easy-to-follow healthy lifestyle supporting your well-being.

- Start with small changes: The DASH diet is a lifestyle change, not a quick fix. Start by making minor changes to your diet and lifestyle, such as swapping processed snacks for whole-grain options or taking a daily walk. Gradually build on these changes to create a sustainable, healthy lifestyle.
- Plan: Planning your meals and snacks can help you stay on track with the DASH diet. Try meal prepping on weekends or planning your meals for the week ahead. This can help you avoid unhealthy choices when you're busy or short on time.
- Emphasize whole, nutrient-dense foods: Choose foods rich in fiber, vitamins, and minerals. Vegetables, Fruits, whole grains, lean proteins, and low-fat dairy products are all great choices on the DASH diet. Aim to include a variety of these foods in your diet each day.
- Limit processed and high-sodium foods: Processed and high-sodium foods can contribute to high blood pressure, heart disease, and other health problems. Limit your intake of these foods and choose healthier alternatives whenever possible.
- Be mindful of portion sizes: Even healthy foods can contribute to weight gain if you overeat them. Pay attention to portion sizes and try to eat slowly and mindfully. This can help you avoid overeating and promote a healthier relationship with food.

- Staying hydrated: Drinking plenty of water is essential for overall well-being and well-being. Limit intake of sugary drinks such as soft drinks and fruit juices and drink at least eight glasses of water a day.

Stay active: The DASH diet emphasizes the importance of physical activity. Important exercise at least 150 minutes a week at moderate intensity and incorporate some strength exercises or with weightlifting or bodyweight exercises.

Food Serving Recommendations for The Dash Diet

Now let's see a list of the recommended foods to follow this diet best. These foods have been selected for their nutritional value, calorie content, and, generally, for how easily you can find them in your favorite supermarket.

- Vegetables: Aim for 4-5 servings per day
- Fruits: Aim for 4-5 servings per day
- Grains (mainly whole grains): Aim for 6-8 servings daily.
- Lean proteins (e.g., poultry, fish, beans, nuts): Aim for six or fewer servings daily.
- Low-fat dairy products (e.g., milk, yogurt, cheese): Aim for 2-3 servings daily.
- Fats and oils (e.g., olive oil, canola oil): Use in moderation
- Sweets and added sugars: Limit your intake.
- Vegetables: Aim for a variety of colors and types, including leafy greens, cruciferous vegetables (e.g., broccoli, cauliflower), and starchy vegetables (e.g., sweet potatoes, corn)
- Fruits: Aim for a variety of colors and types, including berries, citrus fruits, and tropical fruits
- Grains (mainly whole grains): Aim for various whole grains, including brown rice, quinoa, oats, whole-grain bread, and pasta.
- Lean proteins (e.g., poultry, fish, beans, nuts): Choose lean cuts of meat and remove visible fat. Include plant-based protein sources like beans, lentils, and tofu.
- Low-fat dairy products (e.g., milk, yogurt, cheese): Choose low-fat or fat-free options. You can also try non-dairy alternatives like almond milk or soy yogurt.
- Fats and oils (e.g., olive oil, canola oil): Use in moderation, and choose healthier fats like olive oil and avocados.
- Sweets and added sugars: Limit your intake of sweets and added sugars and choose healthier alternatives like fresh fruit or unsweetened yogurt.

What to eat and avoid on the Dash diet

The DASH diet is a healthy diet focusing on whole, nutrient-dense foods and limiting processed and high-sodium foods. To follow the DASH diet, you should eat plenty of fruits, vegetables, lean, whole grains, proteins, and low-fat dairy products. These foods are rich in nutrients like fiber, vitamins, and minerals and can help support overall health and well-being.

It's important to limit or avoid foods high in sodium, like processed meats, canned soups, pre-packaged snacks, sweets, and added sugars, which can contribute to weight gain and other health problems. Alcohol should also be limited, as excessive alcohol consumption can have negative health effects.

To make the DASH diet work for you, it's important to plan your meals and snacks and pay attention to portion sizes. You should also stay hydrated by drinking plenty of water and staying active with regular exercise.

Plan your meals and snack.

Planning your meals and snacks means considering what you will eat ahead rather than deciding on the spot. This can help you make healthier choices and avoid unhealthy options when you're busy or short on time.

To plan your meals and snacks, you can take a few simple steps:

- *Decide what meals and snacks you're going to eat*: Look at your schedule for the upcoming week and decide what meals and snacks you're going to eat. This can help you avoid last-minute decisions that may not be the healthiest. You can also consider what foods you enjoy and which are DASH-friendly to help you plan.
- *Create a grocery list:* Once you've decided what meals and snacks you'll eat, make a grocery list of the foods you'll need to make those meals and snacks. This can help you avoid forgetting key ingredients and simplify grocery shopping. Make sure to include plenty of fresh fruits and vegetables, whole grains, lean proteins, and low-fat dairy products on your list.
- *Prep ingredients in advance:* If possible, you can also prep some ingredients in advance, like cutting up vegetables or marinating chicken. This can help make cooking meals faster and easier when you're short on time. You can also cook meals in advance and store them in the fridge or freezer for later in the week.
- *By planning your meals and snacks*, you can make healthier choices and avoid unhealthy options. This can be especially helpful when following the DASH diet, as it can be easy to reach for processed or high-sodium foods when you're short on time or don't have a plan. Planning your meals and snacks can also save you time and money and help reduce food waste by using ingredients before they spoil.
- Additionally, you can try *meal prepping on the weekends*, preparing several meals or snacks for the week ahead. This can be a great way to ensure healthy options throughout the week, even when busy or on the go.

Decide what meals and snack you're going to eat.

- Look at your schedule: Look at your upcoming week and consider what meals and snacks will work best for your schedule. For example, if you have a busy day on Wednesday, you may want to plan a quick and easy dinner for that night.
- Consider your preferences: Consider the foods you enjoy and what types of meals and snacks you'd like to eat during the week. Plan a taco night or make a healthy burrito bowl if you love

Mexican food. If you enjoy breakfast foods, you could plan to make overnight oats or a veggie-packed frittata for breakfast.

- Plan for variety: Include various foods and flavors in your meal plan. This can help prevent boredom and ensure you get a wide range of nutrients. For example, you could plan to make a vegetarian stir-fry one night, a grilled chicken salad the next, and a seafood dish for another night.
- Check for DASH-friendliness: When planning your meals and snacks, choose DASH-friendly foods. This means focusing on whole, nutrient-dense foods like vegetables, fruits, whole grains, lean proteins, and low-fat dairy products and limiting processed and high-sodium foods.
- Consider leftovers: Planning meals that will provide leftovers can be a great way to save time and reduce food waste. For example, you could plan to make a big pot of chili or soup for several meals.

Create a grocery list.

- Plan your meals and snacks: Before creating your grocery list, plan what meals and snacks you'll be eating for the upcoming week. This will help ensure you have all the necessary ingredients to make healthy, DASH-friendly meals and snacks.
- Include a variety of foods: Make sure to include various foods on your grocery list, including fresh, vegetables and fruits, whole grains, lean proteins and low-fat dairy products. This will help ensure you get a wide range of nutrients and flavors.
- Check your pantry and fridge: Before heading to the store, check your pantry and fridge to see what items you already have. This can help you avoid buying duplicate articles and can help reduce food waste.
- Make a detailed list: Once you've planned your meals and snacks and checked your pantry and fridge, make a detailed list of the items you'll need to buy at the store. Organize the list by category (e.g., produce, dairy, meat) to make shopping easier.
- Consider your budget: As you make your grocery list, consider your budget, and choose items that fit within your means. Look for sales and coupons on healthy items to help save money.
- Shop the perimeter: When at the store, focus on shopping the perimeter, where you'll find fresh produce, lean proteins, and low-fat dairy products. Avoid the inner aisles, where you'll find more processed and high-sodium foods.

Prep ingredients in advance

- Plan your meals and snacks: Before prepping ingredients in advance, plan what meals and snacks you'll be eating for the upcoming week. This will help ensure you have all the necessary ingredients to make healthy, DASH-friendly meals and snacks.
- Choose ingredients to prep: Once you've planned your meals and snacks, choose which ingredients you can prep in advance. This could include chopping vegetables, cooking whole grains or lean proteins, or making a batch of salad dressing or marinade.
- Set aside time: Set aside a specific time to prep ingredients in advance, such as on the weekend or during a less busy weeknight. This will help ensure you have enough time to get everything done.
- Use proper storage containers: Use proper storage containers to keep prepped ingredients fresh. This could include airtight containers for chopped vegetables, cooked grains, or a covered dish for marinated proteins.
- Label containers: Label containers with the date and contents to help keep track of what you've prepped and ensure you use everything before it goes bad.

- Store in the fridge or freezer: Once you've prepped your ingredients, store them in the fridge or freezer until you're ready to use them. This can help make cooking meals faster and easier when you're short on time.

Benefit of the Dash diet

The DASH diet is healthy and can benefit overall health and well-being. The main benefits are for your body and also your mind. This diet will allow you to achieve excellent results; if followed correctly, these results will be short.

Hearth Health
The DASH diet is designed to be low in sodium and high in nutrients beneficial for heart health, such as fiber, potassium, and magnesium. Here's how the DASH diet can help promote heart health:
Reduces blood pressure: heart disease is significantly increased by high blood pressure. The DASH diet is made to be high in potassium and low in sodium, both of which can lower blood pressure. According to studies, adopting the DASH diet can lower blood pressure and the chance of developing heart disease.
Reduces inflammation: Inflammation in the body is linked to various health problems, including heart disease. The DASH diet is rich in anti-inflammatory foods like fruits, whole grains, and vegetables, which can help reduce inflammation and promote heart health.
Enhances cholesterol levels: High "bad" LDL cholesterol levels can raise heart disease risk. The DASH diet is made to be high in fiber and low in saturated fat, which can help lower cholesterol and lower the risk of heart disease.
Promotes healthy blood vessels: Potassium, magnesium, and calcium are some of the minerals in the DASH diet that can help support healthy blood vessels and lower the risk of heart disease.
Lowers the risk of heart disease: It has been demonstrated that adopting the DASH diet will reduce your risk of developing heart disease. The National Heart, Lung, and Blood Institute initially created the DASH diet to lower the risk of heart disease.

Supports weight management.
The DASH diet emphasizes whole, nutrient-dense foods like vegetables. fruits, , and lean proteins while limiting processed and high-calorie foods. Here's how the DASH diet can support weight management:
Reduces calorie intake: The DASH diet can help reduce calorie intake by focusing on whole, nutrient-dense foods. Depending on your goals, this can lead to weight loss or maintenance.
Increases satiety: The fiber and protein in the DASH diet can help increase feelings of fullness and reduce hunger. This can help prevent overeating and support weight management.
Supports healthy metabolism: The nutrients in the DASH diet, such as magnesium and calcium, can help support healthy metabolism and energy production. This can help support weight management by keeping your body functioning correctly.
Reduces the risk of obesity: Following the DASH diet can help reduce the risk of obesity, which is a significant risk factor for many chronic diseases. Maintaining a healthy weight can reduce your risk of developing health problems like heart disease, diabetes, and certain types of cancer.
Encourages healthy habits: The DASH diet emphasizes healthy habits like regular physical activity, which can help support weight management. By incorporating healthy habits into your lifestyle, you can make sustainable changes that support long-term weight management.

Reduce Inflammation
Inflammation is the body's natural response to injury or infection. Still, chronic inflammation can contribute to various health problems, including heart disease, diabetes, and cancer. The DASH diet is rich in anti-

inflammatory foods like fruits and vegetables, which can help reduce inflammation. Here's how the DASH diet can reduce inflammation:

Provides antioxidants: Antioxidants are nutrients that can help protect the body from damage caused by inflammation. The DASH diet is rich in antioxidant-rich foods.

Reduces intake of pro-inflammatory foods: The DASH diet limits or eliminates processed and high-fat foods, which are pro-inflammatory. By reducing the input of these foods, the DASH diet can help reduce inflammation in the body.

Provides omega-3 fatty acids: Omega-3 fatty acids are a type of fat that can help reduce inflammation in the body. The DASH diet includes foods like fatty fish, nuts, and seeds, which are good sources of omega-3 fatty acids.

Promotes healthy gut bacteria: The DASH diet is fiber-rich, which can help promote beneficial gut bacteria. Healthy gut bacteria can help reduce inflammation by supporting the immune system.

Improves Digestion

The DASH diet is high in fiber, which can help support healthy digestion and prevent constipation. Here's how the DASH diet can improve digestion:

Provides fiber: Fiber is a type of carbohydrate that is not digested by the body. Instead, it passes through the digestive system, adding bulk to stool and promoting regular bowel movements.

Supports gut health: Fiber also acts as a prebiotic, which helps promote healthy gut bacteria growth. Beneficial gut bacteria are essential for healthy digestion, as they help break down food and absorb nutrients. By eating a variety of fiber-rich foods, you can support healthy gut bacteria and improve digestion.

Reduces constipation: A common digestive problem that can cause discomfort and bloating. The fiber in the DASH diet can help prevent constipation by adding bulk to stool and promoting regular bowel movements.

Supports weight management: Maintaining a healthy weight is essential for digestive health. Excess weight can pressure the digestive system and contribute to problems like heartburn and acid reflux. The DASH diet can support weight management by promoting healthy eating habits and providing nutrient-dense, low-calorie foods.

Reduces risk of digestive problems: Digestive problems like irritable bowel syndrome (IBS) and inflammatory bowel disease (IBD) are linked to chronic inflammation in the gut. By reducing inflammation in the body through an anti-inflammatory diet like the DASH diet, you can reduce the risk of digestive problems.

Support Brain

The DASH diet is rich in essential nutrients for brain health, such as omega-3 fatty acids, antioxidants, and B vitamins. Here's how the DASH diet can support brain health:

Provides omega-3 fatty acids: Omega-3 fatty acids are a type of fat important for brain health, and they can help improve cognitive function, reduce inflammation in the brain, and support healthy brain aging. The DASH diet includes foods like fatty fish, nuts, and seeds, which are good sources of omega-3 fatty acids.

Provides antioxidants: Antioxidants are nutrients that can help protect the brain from damage caused by inflammation and oxidative stress.

Provides B vitamins: B vitamins are essential for brain function and development. The DASH diet includes foods like whole grains, leafy greens, and low-fat dairy products, which are good sources of B vitamins.

Reduces the risk of cognitive decline: Following the DASH diet has been shown to reduce mental decline risk, a common problem in aging adults. By providing essential nutrients for brain health and reducing the risk of chronic diseases like heart disease and diabetes, the DASH diet can support healthy brain aging.

Supports overall health: The DASH diet promotes overall health and well-being, which can indirectly support brain health. The DASH diet can support brain health and cognitive function by reducing the risk of chronic diseases and promoting healthy habits like regular physical activity.

Boost Energy

The DASH diet is rich in nutrients supporting healthy energy levels, such as complex carbohydrates, B vitamins, and iron. Here's how the DASH diet can boost energy:

Provides complex carbohydrates: Complex carbohydrates are a type of carbohydrate that is digested slowly, providing a steady source of energy over time. The DASH diet includes whole grains, fruits, vegetables, and good complex carbohydrates seeds.

Provides B vitamins: B vitamins are essential for energy production and can help support healthy energy levels. The DASH diet includes foods like whole grains, leafy greens, and low-fat dairy products, which are good sources of B vitamins.

Provides iron: Iron is essential for healthy energy levels, as it helps transport oxygen throughout the body. The DASH diet includes foods like lean meats, beans, and leafy greens, which are good sources of iron.

Reduces intake of processed foods: Processed foods are often high in added sugars and unhealthy fats, contributing to energy crashes and fatigue. By reducing the input of these foods and focusing on nutrient-dense, whole foods, the DASH diet can help support healthy energy levels.

Encourages healthy habits: The DASH diet emphasizes healthy habits like regular physical activity, which can help boost energy levels. By incorporating healthy habits into your lifestyle, you can make sustainable changes that support long-term energy levels.

What nutrient do I need to regulate?

To maintain good health, it's essential to regulate a variety of nutrients in your diet. Some critical nutrients you may need to regulate include sodium, potassium, calcium, magnesium, and fiber.

Although salt is a necessary nutrient, overeating can raise blood pressure and increase the risk of heart disease. Therefore, the DASH diet advises keeping salt intake to a maximum of 2,300 mg daily. In addition, restricting the consumption of processed and packaged foods is essential to reduce sodium intake, which is often high in sodium. Instead, focus on cooking meals from scratch using whole, unprocessed foods.

Potassium is essential for healthy blood pressure and heart function. The DASH diet recommends consuming 4,700 milligrams of potassium per day, which can be achieved by eating various fruits, vegetables, and low-fat dairy products. Therefore, increase your potassium intake, incorporate more fruits and vegetables into your diet, and choose low-fat dairy products like milk, yogurt, and cheese.

Calcium is essential for healthy bones and teeth. The DASH diet includes low-fat dairy products as a source of calcium. To ensure adequate calcium intake, have low-fat dairy products like milk, yogurt, and cheese. Suppose you are lactose intolerant or avoid dairy. You can also get calcium from fortified plant-based milk, leafy greens, and nuts.

Magnesium is essential for healthy nerve and muscle function. The DASH diet includes whole grains, nuts, and seeds as sources of magnesium. To increase magnesium intake, incorporate more whole grains like brown rice, whole wheat bread and quinoa into your diet, and choose nuts and seeds as a snack.

Fiber is crucial for a healthy digestive system, and in addition, it can lower the chance of developing heart disease and chronic diseases such as diabetes. Fruits, vegetables, and whole grains are among the foods high in fiber that are part of the DASH diet... The DASH diet is high in fiber-rich foods like fruits, vegetables, and whole grains. To increase fiber intake, incorporate more fruits, vegetables, and whole grains into your diet. In addition, choose snacks like nuts and seeds instead of processed snacks.

By regulating these nutrients through a balanced diet like the DASH diet, you can support overall health and reduce the risk of chronic diseases. Remember, focusing on making sustainable, long-term changes to your diet and lifestyle is essential to achieve the best results.

Focusing on overall dietary patterns and healthy lifestyle habits is essential to regulate these critical nutrients. The DASH diet promotes overall health and well-being by emphasizing nutrient-dense, whole foods and healthy lifestyle habits like regular physical activity.

- Incorporate a variety of fruits and vegetables into your diet: Vegetables and Fruits are rich in vitamins, minerals, and fiber and can help support overall health. Aim to incorporate various colors and types of vegetables and fruits into your diet to ensure you get a range of nutrients.
- Select whole grains over refined grains since they are fiber-rich and support a healthy digestive system. Examples of whole grains are brown rice, quinoa, and whole wheat bread. To maximize the nutritional value of your diet, choose whole grains over refined grains like white bread and pasta.
- Choose lean protein sources: Lean protein sources like chicken, fish, and legumes can help support muscle growth and repair. Choose lean protein sources over fatty meats like beef and pork, which can increase the risk of heart disease.
- Limit added sugars and unhealthy fats: Added sugars and unhealthy fats like saturated and trans fats can contribute to chronic diseases like heart disease and diabetes. Limit your intake of these foods and focus on nutrient-dense, whole foods instead.
- Engage in regular physical activity: Regular physical activity is essential for overall health and well-being. Aim for at least 2 hours of moderate or 1 - 75 minutes of vigorous-intensity exercise per week.
- By following these tips and incorporating the principles of the DASH diet into your lifestyle, you can support overall health and reduce the risk of chronic diseases. Remember, focusing on making sustainable, long-term changes to your diet and lifestyle is essential to achieve the best results.

The DASH diet is a balanced and flexible diet that promotes overall health and reduces the risk of chronic diseases. Focusing on nutrient-dense, whole foods and healthy lifestyle habits can support your body and mind and achieve long-term success.

Remember, making sustainable changes to your diet and lifestyle is critical to achieving the best results. It's essential to be patient and persistent and to focus on progress rather than perfection. Small, incremental changes can increase over time and significantly improve your health.

Suppose you're considering starting the DASH diet. In that case, it's essential to talk to your healthcare provider first, especially if you have any underlying health conditions or are taking medication. They can help you determine if the DASH diet is proper for you and provide guidance on how to follow it safely and effectively.

Incorporating the principles of the DASH diet into your lifestyle can be a decisive step toward achieving optimal health and well-being. By caring for your body and mind through balanced nutrition and healthy habits, you can enjoy a happier, healthier life for years.

Dash diet FAQ

1. What does DASH stand for?

The Dietary Approach to Stop Hypertension is known as DASH. The DASH diet was created by the National Institutes of Health to assist lower blood pressure and lowering the risk of heart disease.

1. What aims does the DASH diet pursue?

The DASH diet promotes overall health and reduces the risk of chronic diseases like heart disease, stroke, and diabetes. The DASH diet is designed to be a balanced and flexible eating plan emphasizing nutrient-dense, whole foods and healthy lifestyle habits like regular physical activity.

1. What foods should I eat on the DASH diet?

The DASH diet emphasizes a variety of nutrient-dense, vegetables, whole foods like fruits, whole grains, lean protein sources, and low-fat dairy products. Examples of foods to include on the DASH diet include:

- Fruits like apples, bananas, oranges, and berries
- Vegetables like broccoli, carrots, spinach, and tomatoes
- Brown rice, quinoa, and whole wheat bread are examples of whole grains.
- Sources of lean protein, including poultry, fish, and beans
- dairy items with low fat, including milk, yogurt, and cheese.

1. What foods should I avoid on the DASH diet?

The DASH diet recommends limiting the intake of processed and packaged foods and foods high in sodium, saturated fat and added sugars. Examples of foods to limit or avoid on the DASH diet include:
- Processed and packaged foods like chips, crackers, and frozen dinners
- Foods high in sodium, like canned soups, cured meats, and fast food.
- Fatty meats like beef and pork
- Foods high in added sugars, like candy, soda, and desserts

1. Is the DASH diet effective for weight loss?

The DASH diet can effectively lose weight, especially with regular physical activity and healthy lifestyle habits. In addition, the DASH diet emphasizes nutrient-dense, low-calorie foods like vegetables, fruits, and whole grains, which can help you feel full and satisfied while supporting weight loss.

1. How much sodium should I consume on the DASH diet?

The DASH diet suggests keeping sodium consumption to a maximum of 2,300 milligrams, or 1,500 milligrams for people with high blood pressure. In addition, the DASH diet calls for limiting the consumption of packaged and processed foods and preparing meals from scratch using whole, unprocessed ingredients.

1. Does the DASH diet allow alcohol consumption?

Moderate alcohol consumption can be included in a healthy diet, but excessive alcohol consumption should be avoided. The DASH diet recommends limiting alcohol intake to 1/2 drink per day for women and no more than one drink per day for men.

1. Is the DASH diet suitable for vegetarians or vegans?

The DASH diet can be modified to accommodate a vegetarian or vegan lifestyle by incorporating plant-based protein sources like beans, nuts, and seeds. However, to ensure adequate protein intake on a vegetarian or vegan DASH diet, it's essential to include a variety of protein sources in your diet and to consider supplementing with vitamin B12.

1. How can I make the DASH diet more affordable?

To make the DASH diet more affordable, focus on buying in-season produce, buying in bulk, and cooking meals from scratch using whole, unprocessed foods. It's also important to plan meals and snacks in advance to avoid impulse purchases and food waste.

1. Can children follow the DASH diet?

The DASH diet can be adapted for children by adjusting portions and incorporating appropriate foods. The DASH diet emphasizes nutrient-dense, whole foods that can support healthy growth and development in children while reducing the risk of chronic diseases like obesity and type 2 diabetes.

1. Can the DASH diet be followed long-term?

Yes, the DASH diet is designed to be a long-term eating plan that can be followed for a lifetime to support overall health and well-being. The DASH diet emphasizes balanced nutrition and healthy lifestyle habits that can help you feel your best and reduce the risk of chronic diseases like heart disease and diabetes.

1. Is the DASH diet safe for everyone?

Even though the DASH diet is generally safe for most individuals, it is imperative to see your doctor before beginning it, especially if you have any underlying medical conditions or are taking medication. Your health care provider can help you determine whether if the DASH diet is proper for you and provide guidance on how to follow it safely and effectively.

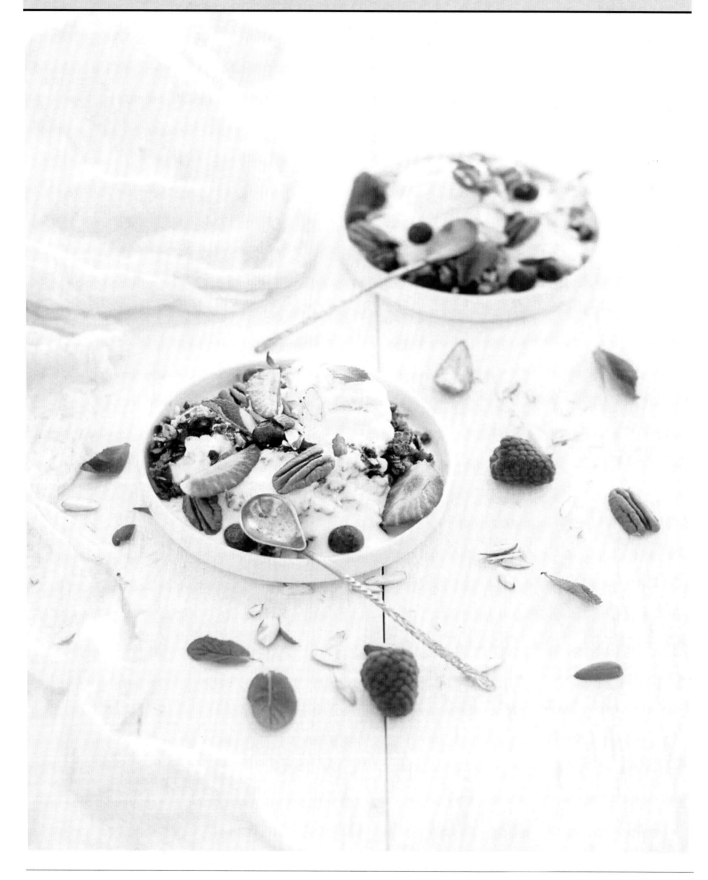

Greek Yogurt Parfait with Berries and Granola

Preparation time: 10 minutes **Servings:** 2

Ingredients:

- 1 cup of plain non-fat Greek yogurt
- 1 cup of mixed berries (such as strawberries, blueberries, or raspberries)
- 1/2 cup of low-sugar granola
- 1 tablespoon of honey (optional)

Instructions:

1. Rinse the mixed berries under running water and chop them if necessary.
2. Add a layer of Greek yogurt in two separate serving glasses or jars.
3. Add a layer of mixed berries on top of the yogurt.
4. Sprinkle granola over the mixed berries to form another layer.
5. Repeat the layers until the glasses are filled, making sure to end with a layer of granola on top.
6. Drizzle honey over the top layer of granola (if using).
7. Chill the parfait in the refrigerator for 30 minutes to 1 hour.
8. Serve and enjoy!

Nutritional Values: Calories: 205 Total Fat: 2 g Saturated Fat: 0 g Cholesterol: 3 mg Sodium: 76 mg
Total Carbohydrate: 36 g Dietary Fiber: 4 g Total Sugars: 18 g Protein: 17 g

Berry and Spinach Smoothie Bowl

Preparation time: 5 minutes **Servings:** 2

Ingredients:

- 2 cups of fresh spinach leaves
- 1 ripe banana, sliced.
- 1 cup of mixed frozen berries (such as strawberries, blueberries, and raspberries)
- 1/2 cup of low-fat milk or unsweetened almond milk
- 1/2 cup of plain non-fat Greek yogurt
- 1 tablespoon of honey (optional)
- 1/4 cup of low-sugar granola
- 2 tablespoons of chia seeds (optional)

Instructions:

1. Add the spinach leaves, sliced banana, mixed frozen berries, milk, and Greek yogurt in a blender.
2. Blend the ingredients until smooth and creamy.
3. If desired, add honey to sweeten the smoothie taste.
4. Pour the smoothie into two serving bowls.
5. Top each bowl with a sprinkle of granola and chia seeds if using.
6. Serve and enjoy!

Nutritional Values: Calories: 210 Total Fat: 3 g Saturated Fat: 1 g Cholesterol: 6 mg Sodium: 78 mg Total Carbohydrate: 39 g Dietary Fiber: 7 g Total Sugars: 23 g Protein: 10 g

Veggie Omelet with Spinach

Preparation time: 10 minutes **Cooking Time:** 10 minutes **Servings:** 2

Ingredients:

- 4 large eggs
- 1 cup of fresh spinach, chopped.
- 1 medium tomato, diced.
- 1/2 cup of mushrooms, sliced.
- 1/4 tsp of salt
- 1/8 tsp of black pepper
- 1 tbsp. of extra-virgin olive oil
- 1/4 cup of low-fat shredded cheese

Instructions:

1. In a medium bowl, beat the eggs with salt and black pepper until well combined.
2. Heat a large non-stick skillet over medium heat. Add the olive oil and swirl to coat the bottom of the skillet.
3. Add the chopped spinach, mushrooms, and diced tomatoes to the skillet. Cook, frequently stirring, for about 5 minutes or until the vegetables are tender and the excess moisture has evaporated.

4. Reduce the heat to medium-low and pour the beaten eggs over the vegetables. Tilt the skillet to ensure the eggs cover the entire surface of the skillet.

5. Sprinkle the shredded cheese over the omelet and cover it with a lid. Cook for 3-5 minutes until the eggs are set and the cheese is melted.

6. Fold the omelet in half using a spatula and slide it onto a serving plate. Serve hot.

Nutritional Values: Calories: 227kcal Total Fat: 16g Saturated Fat: 5g Cholesterol: 347mg Sodium: 454mg Total Carbohydrate: 6g Dietary Fiber: 1g Sugar: 3g Protein: 16g

Sweet Potato and Black Bean Breakfast Burrito

Preparation time: 20 minutes **Cooking Time:** 20 minutes **Servings:** 4

Ingredients:

- 2 medium sweet potatoes peeled and diced.
- 1 can of black beans, drained and rinsed.
- 1 red bell pepper, diced.
- 1/2 red onion, diced.
- 1 tablespoon of olive oil
- 1 teaspoon of ground cumin
- 1/2 teaspoon of chili powder
- Salt and pepper, to taste
- 4 whole wheat tortillas
- 4 large eggs
- 1/2 cup of shredded low-fat cheddar cheese
- Salsa, for serving (optional)

Instructions:

1. Preheat the oven to 400°F (200°C).

2. Mix the sweet potato, black beans, red bell pepper, red onion, olive oil, ground cumin, chili powder, salt, and pepper in a large bowl.

3. Spread the mixture in a single layer on a baking sheet and roast in the oven for 20 minutes or until the sweet potatoes are tender.

4. While the sweet potato mixture is roasting, heat a non-stick skillet over medium heat.

5. Crack the eggs into the skillet and cook them to your preferred level of doneness.

6. Warm the whole wheat tortillas in the microwave or on a skillet.

7. To assemble the burritos, divide the sweet potato mixture, scrambled eggs, and shredded cheese evenly among the four tortillas.

8. Fold the tortillas up into a burrito shape.

9. Serve with salsa, if desired.

Nutritional Values: Calories: 375 Total Fat: 13 g Saturated Fat: 4 g Cholesterol: 213 mg Sodium: 450 mg Total Carbohydrate: 47 g Dietary Fiber: 12 g Total Sugars: 7 g Protein: 21 g

Broccoli and Feta Frittata

Preparation time: 10 minutes **Cooking Time:** 20 minutes **Servings:** 4

Ingredients:

- 8 large eggs
- 1/2 cup of crumbled feta cheese
- 1 head of broccoli, chopped into small florets.
- 1/2 red onion, diced.
- 1 tablespoon of olive oil
- Salt and pepper, to taste

Instructions:

1. Preheat the oven to 350°F (180°C).

2. In a large bowl, whisk the eggs until frothy.

3. Add the crumbled feta cheese to the bowl and mix well.

4. In a 10-inch oven-safe skillet, heat the olive oil over medium heat.

5. Add the chopped broccoli and red onion to the skillet and sauté for 5-7 minutes until the vegetables are tender.

6. Pour the egg mixture over the sautéed vegetables.

7. Cook for 3-4 minutes, stirring gently until the edges are set.

8. Transfer the skillet to the preheated oven and bake for 10-12 minutes or until the frittata is set in the center.
9. Remove from the oven and let it cool for a few minutes.
10. Slice the frittata into wedges and serve.

Nutritional Values: Calories: 209 Total Fat: 15 g Saturated Fat: 5 g Cholesterol: 370 mg Sodium: 361 mg Total Carbohydrate: 6 g Dietary Fiber: 2 g Total Sugars: 2 g Protein: 15 g

Avocado Toast with Poached Egg

Preparation time: 10 minutes **Cooking Time:** 10 minutes **Servings:** 2
Ingredients:

- 2 slices of whole-grain bread
- 1 ripe avocado
- 4 cherry tomatoes, halved.
- 2 large eggs
- 1/4 tsp of salt
- 1/8 tsp of black pepper
- 1 tsp of white vinegar
- 1 tbsp. of chopped fresh parsley.

Instructions:

1. Toast the slices of bread until golden brown.
2. Cut the avocado in half and remove the pit. Scoop out the flesh into a bowl and mash it with a fork until smooth. Season with salt and black pepper to taste.
3. Top each slice of toast with the mashed avocado and halved cherry tomatoes.
4. Bring 2 inches of water to a simmer over medium heat in a medium pot. Add the white vinegar and stir.
5. Crack one egg into a small cup or ramekin. Using a spoon, create a whirlpool in the simmering water and gently slide the egg into the center of the vortex. Poach the egg for 2-3 minutes or until the white is set and the yolk is still runny.
6. Use a slotted spoon to carefully remove the poached egg from the water and place it on top of one of the avocado toasts. Repeat the same process with the second egg.

7. Sprinkle the chopped parsley over the avocado toast with poached eggs and serve immediately.

Nutritional Values: Calories: 236kcal Total Fat: 14g Saturated Fat: 3g Cholesterol: 185mg Sodium: 316mg Total Carbohydrate: 19g Dietary Fiber: 7g Sugar: 2g Protein: 11g

Low-Fat Breakfast Quesadilla

Preparation time: 10 minutes **Cooking Time:** 10 minutes **Servings:** 2
Ingredients:

- 2 whole wheat tortillas
- 4 large eggs
- 1/2 cup of canned black beans, drained and rinsed.
- 1/2 red bell pepper, diced.
- 1/2 red onion, diced.
- 1/2 cup of shredded low-fat cheddar cheese
- 1 tablespoon of olive oil
- Salt and pepper, to taste

Instructions:

1. In a non-stick skillet, heat the olive oil over medium heat.
2. Add the diced red bell pepper and red onion to the skillet and sauté for 5 minutes until tender.
3. Add the black beans to the skillet and cook for 1-2 minutes until heated.
4. Crack the eggs into a bowl and whisk them together.
5. Pour the eggs into the skillet with the vegetables and cook, occasionally stirring, until the eggs are scrambled and cooked through.
6. Divide the egg mixture into two portions and place each piece onto a tortilla.
7. Top each tortilla with 1/4 cup of shredded low-fat cheddar cheese.
8. Fold the tortillas in half to form a quesadilla.
9. Heat the quesadillas in a skillet over medium heat until the cheese is melted, and the tortillas are crispy.

10. Slice the quesadillas into wedges and serve.

Nutritional Values: Calories: 395 Total Fat: 19 g Saturated Fat: 6 g Cholesterol: 380 mg Sodium: 605 mg Total Carbohydrate: 33 g Dietary Fiber: 11 g Total Sugars: 2 g Protein: 27 g

Steel-Cut Oatmeal with Apples

Preparation time: 5 minutes **Cooking Time:** 25 minutes **Servings:** 4

Ingredients:

- 1 cup of steel-cut oats
- 4 cups of water
- 2 medium apples peeled and diced.
- 1 teaspoon of ground cinnamon
- 1/4 cup of chopped walnuts
- 2 tablespoons of honey (optional)
- 1/2 cup of low-fat milk or unsweetened almond milk (optional)

Instructions:

1. In a medium-sized saucepan, bring the water to a boil.
2. Add the steel-cut oats to the boiling water and reduce the heat to low.
3. Simmer the oats, occasionally stirring, for 20-25 minutes or until the oats are tender and the mixture has thickened.
4. While the oats are cooking, mix the diced apples and ground cinnamon in a small bowl.
5. When the oats are cooked, stir in the apple mixture, and cook for 3-5 minutes until the apples are softened.
6. Remove the oats from the heat and stir in the chopped walnuts.
7. If desired, add honey to sweeten the oatmeal to taste.
8. Serve the oatmeal in individual bowls, and if desired, top it with a splash of low-fat milk or unsweetened almond milk.

Nutritional Values: Calories: 225 Total Fat: 7 g Saturated Fat: 1 g Cholesterol: 0 mg Sodium: 7 mg Total Carbohydrate: 37 g Dietary Fiber: 6 g Total Sugars: 14 g Protein: 7 g

Smoked Salmon and Cucumber

Preparation time: 10 minutes **Servings:** 2

Ingredients:

- 2 slices of whole-grain bread
- 2 ounces of smoked salmon
- 1/2 English cucumber, sliced.
- 2 tablespoons of low-fat cream cheese
- 1 tablespoon of chopped fresh dill.
- Salt and pepper, to taste
- Lemon wedges for serving (optional)

Instructions:

1. Toast the slices of whole-grain bread until crispy.
2. Mix the low-fat cream cheese and chopped fresh dill in a small bowl until well combined.
3. Spread the cream cheese mixture onto the toasted bread slices.
4. Top each bread slice with slices of smoked salmon and sliced cucumber.
5. Season with salt and pepper to taste.
6. Serve with lemon wedges on the side, if desired.

Nutritional Values: Calories: 183 Total Fat: 6 g Saturated Fat: 2 g Cholesterol: 20 mg Sodium: 418 mg Total Carbohydrate: 19 g Dietary Fiber: 4 g Total Sugars: 3 g Protein: 16 g

Whole-Grain Banana Pancakes

Preparation time: 15 minutes **Cooking Time:** 15 minutes **Servings:** 4

Ingredients:

- 1 cup of whole-grain flour
- 1 tbsp. of baking powder
- 1/4 tsp of salt
- 1 ripe banana, mashed.
- 1 cup of low-fat milk
- 1 large egg
- 1 tbsp. of canola oil
- 2 tbsp. of natural peanut butter
- 2 tbsp. of honey

Instructions:

1. Whisk together the whole-grain flour, baking powder, and salt in a large bowl.

2. Whisk together the mashed banana, low-fat milk, egg, and canola oil in a separate bowl until smooth.

3. Add the wet ingredients to the dry ingredients and stir until well combined.

4. Heat a large non-stick skillet or griddle over medium-high heat. Use a ladle or measuring cup to pour the pancake batter onto the skillet, making 4–5-inch pancakes.

5. Cook the pancakes for 2-3 minutes or until bubbles form on the surface and the edges start to look dry. Flip the pancakes and cook for 1-2 minutes or until golden brown.

6. Serve the whole-grain banana pancakes with a dollop of natural peanut butter and a drizzle of honey on top.

Nutritional Values: Calories: 276kcal Total Fat: 9g Saturated Fat: 1g Cholesterol: 41mg Sodium: 456mg Total Carbohydrate: 44g Dietary Fiber: 4g Sugar: 19g Protein: 8g

Cottage Cheese and Berry Breakfast Bowl

Preparation time: 5 minutes **Servings:** 2
Ingredients:
- 1 cup of low-fat cottage cheese
- 1 cup of mixed berries (such as strawberries, blueberries, or raspberries)
- 1/4 cup of chopped walnuts
- 2 tablespoons of honey (optional)

Instructions:
1. Rinse the mixed berries under running water and chop them if necessary.

2. In two separate serving bowls, add a layer of low-fat cottage cheese.

3. Add a layer of mixed berries on top of the cottage cheese.

4. Sprinkle chopped walnuts over the mixed berries to form another layer.

5. If desired, drizzle honey over the top of the bowl.

6. Serve and enjoy!

Nutritional Values: Calories: 205 Total Fat: 7 g Saturated Fat: 1 g Cholesterol: 7 mg Sodium: 423

mg
Total Carbohydrate: 23 g Dietary Fiber: 4 g Total Sugars: 18 g Protein: 16 g

Chia Seed Pudding with Almond Milk

Preparation time: 5 minutes **Cooking Time:** 0 minutes (refrigeration time required) **Servings:** 2
Ingredients:
- 1/4 cup of chia seeds
- 1 cup of unsweetened almond milk
- 1 tbsp. of honey
- 1/2 tsp of vanilla extract
- 1 cup of fresh mixed berries (such as strawberries, blueberries, and raspberries)

Instructions:
1. In a medium bowl, whisk together the chia seeds, unsweetened almond milk, honey, and vanilla extract until well combined.

2. Let the mixture rest for 5 minutes, then whisk again to prevent clumping.

3. Cover the bowl with plastic wrap and refrigerate for at least 2 hours or overnight.

4. Before serving, divide the chia seed pudding into two bowls or glasses.

5. Top each bowl or glass with a cup of fresh mixed berries.

6. Serve the chia seed pudding with almond milk and fresh fruit immediately.

Nutritional Values: Calories: 182kcal Total Fat: 7g Saturated Fat: 1g Cholesterol: 0mg Sodium: 91mg Total Carbohydrate: 25g Dietary Fiber: 12g Sugar: 10g Protein: 6g

Baked Eggs with Cherry Tomatoes and Herbs

Preparation time: 10 minutes **Cooking Time:** 20 minutes **Servings:** 2
Ingredients:
- 4 large eggs
- 1 cup of cherry tomatoes, halved.
- 1/4 cup of chopped fresh herbs (such as basil, parsley, or chives)

- 1 tablespoon of olive oil
- Salt and pepper, to taste

Instructions:
1. Preheat the oven to 350°F (180°C).
2. Grease a baking dish with olive oil.
3. Spread the cherry tomatoes out in the baking dish.
4. Crack the eggs over the top of the cherry tomatoes, taking care not to break the yolks.
5. Sprinkle the chopped fresh herbs over the top of the eggs and tomatoes.
6. Season with salt and pepper to taste.
7. Bake in the oven for 15-20 minutes or until the eggs are set.
8. Remove from the oven and let it cool for a few minutes.
9. Divide the baked eggs and cherry tomatoes into two equal portions and serve.

Nutritional Values: Calories: 185 Total Fat: 14 g Saturated Fat: 3 g Cholesterol: 327 mg Sodium: 127 mg Total Carbohydrate: 4 g Dietary Fiber: 1 g Total Sugars: 2 g Protein: 12 g

Peanut Butter and Banana Smoothie

Preparation time: 5 minutes **Servings:** 1
Ingredients:
- 1 ripe banana peeled and sliced.
- 1 tablespoon of natural peanut butter
- 1/2 cup of unsweetened almond milk
- 1/4 teaspoon of ground cinnamon
- 1/2 teaspoon of honey (optional)
- 1/2 cup of ice cubes

Instructions:
1. Add the sliced banana, natural peanut butter, unsweetened almond milk, ground cinnamon, honey (if using), and ice cubes to a blender.
2. Blend all ingredients until smooth and creamy.
3. Pour the smoothie into a glass.
4. Serve immediately and enjoy!

Nutritional Values: Calories: 220 Total Fat: 9 g Saturated Fat: 1 g Cholesterol: 0 mg Sodium: 150

mg
Total Carbohydrate: 31 g Dietary Fiber: 4 g Total Sugars: 16 g Protein: 7 g

Blueberry and Almond Butter Overnight Oats

Preparation time: 5 minutes **Cooking Time:** 0 minutes (overnight) **Servings:** 2
Ingredients:
- 1 cup of rolled oats.
- 1 cup of unsweetened almond milk
- 1/2 cup of fresh blueberries
- 2 tablespoons of almond butter
- 1 tablespoon of chia seeds
- 1/2 teaspoon of vanilla extract
- 1/2 teaspoon of ground cinnamon
- 1 tablespoon of honey (optional)

Instructions:
1. Add the rolled oats, unsweetened almond milk, almond butter, chia seeds, vanilla extract, and ground cinnamon in a medium-sized mixing bowl.
2. Mix all the ingredients until well combined.
3. Divide the oat mixture into two airtight jars or containers.
4. Top each container with fresh blueberries.
5. Cover the jars and refrigerate overnight.
6. Remove the jars from the refrigerator in the morning and stir the oats.
7. If desired, drizzle honey over the top of each jar.
8. Serve and enjoy!

Nutritional Values: Calories: 295 Total Fat: 13 g Saturated Fat: 1 g Cholesterol: 0 mg Sodium: 83 mg
Total Carbohydrate: 38 g Dietary Fiber: 9 g Total Sugars: 8 g Protein: 9 g

Quinoa Breakfast Bowl

Preparation time: 15 minutes **Cooking Time:** 30 minutes **Servings:** 2
Ingredients:
- 1 medium sweet potato, peeled and diced into small cubes.

- 1 tbsp. of olive oil
- 1/2 tsp of paprika
- Salt and black pepper, to taste
- 1/2 cup of quinoa, rinsed.
- 1 cup of low-sodium chicken broth
- 1 ripe avocado, sliced.
- 2 large eggs poached or fried.
- 1/4 cup of chopped fresh parsley.

Instructions:

1. Preheat the oven to 400°F (200°C). Line a baking sheet with parchment paper.
2. Toss the diced sweet potato in a medium bowl with olive oil, paprika, salt, and black pepper until well coated.
3. Spread the sweet potato cubes in a single layer on the prepared baking sheet.
4. Roast the sweet potatoes in the oven for 25-30 minutes or until tender and lightly browned.
5. In a medium saucepan, combine the rinsed quinoa and low-sodium chicken broth. Bring the mixture to a boil over medium-high heat, then reduce the heat to low and cover the saucepan.
6. Simmer the quinoa for 15-20 minutes or until all the liquid has been absorbed and the quinoa is tender.
7. To assemble the quinoa breakfast bowls, divide the cooked quinoa between two bowls.
8. Top each bowl with half the roasted sweet potatoes, sliced avocado, and a poached or fried egg.
9. Garnish each bowl with chopped fresh parsley and serve immediately.

Nutritional Values: Calories: 478kcal Total Fat: 26g Saturated Fat: 4g Cholesterol: 186mg Sodium: 215mg Total Carbohydrate: 47g Dietary Fiber: 10g Sugar: 5g Protein: 18g

Low-Fat Breakfast Wrap

Preparation time: 10 minutes **Cooking Time:** 10 minutes **Servings:** 2
Ingredients:

- 4 large eggs
- 2 whole wheat tortillas
- 1/2 red bell pepper, diced.
- 1/2 zucchini, diced.
- 1/2 yellow onion, diced.
- 1 tablespoon of olive oil
- Salt and pepper, to taste

Instructions:

1. In a non-stick skillet, heat the olive oil over medium heat.
2. Add the diced red bell pepper, zucchini, and yellow onion to the skillet and sauté for 5 minutes until tender.
3. Crack the eggs into a bowl and whisk them together.
4. Pour the eggs into the skillet with the vegetables and cook, occasionally stirring, until the eggs are scrambled and cooked through.
5. Divide the egg mixture into two portions and place each piece onto a tortilla.
6. Roll up the tortillas to form wraps.
7. Heat the wraps in a skillet over medium heat for 1-2 minutes on each side until heated.
8. Slice the wraps in half and serve.

Nutritional Values: Calories: 301 Total Fat: 13 g Saturated Fat: 3 g Cholesterol: 372 mg Sodium: 377 mg Total Carbohydrate: 26 g Dietary Fiber: 5 g Total Sugars: 5 g Protein: 19 g

Spinach and Mushroom Breakfast Skillet

Preparation time: 10 minutes **Cooking Time:** 15 minutes **Servings:** 2
Ingredients:

- 4 large eggs
- 1 cup of sliced mushrooms
- 2 cups of fresh spinach leaves
- 1/2 yellow onion, diced.
- 1 garlic clove, minced.
- 1 tablespoon of olive oil
- Salt and pepper, to taste

Instructions:

1. In a non-stick skillet, heat the olive oil over medium heat.
2. Add the diced yellow onion to the skillet and sauté for 2-3 minutes until translucent.
3. Add the minced garlic to the skillet and sauté for 1-2 minutes until fragrant.
4. Add the sliced mushrooms to the skillet and cook for 3-4 minutes until they have released their liquid and are tender.
5. Add the fresh spinach leaves to the skillet and cook, occasionally stirring, for 2-3 minutes until they have wilted.
6. Crack the eggs into the skillet and cook, stirring occasionally, until they are scrambled and cooked through.
7. Season with salt and pepper to taste.
8. Divide the breakfast skillet into two equal portions and serve.

Nutritional Values: Calories: 206 Total Fat: 14 g Saturated Fat: 3 g Cholesterol: 327 mg Sodium: 168 mg Total Carbohydrate: 7 g Dietary Fiber: 2 g Total Sugars: 2 g Protein: 15 g

Low-Fat Yogurt and Fruit Smoothie

Preparation time: 5 minutes **Cooking Time:** 0 minutes **Servings:** 2
Ingredients:

- 1 cup of low-fat plain yogurt
- 1/2 cup of unsweetened almond milk
- 1 ripe banana peeled and sliced.
- 1 cup of mixed berries (such as strawberries, blueberries, or raspberries)
- 1 tablespoon of honey (optional)

Instructions:

1. Add low-fat plain yogurt, unsweetened almond milk, sliced banana, and mixed berries in a blender.
2. Blend all the ingredients until smooth and creamy.
3. If desired, drizzle honey over the top of the smoothie.
4. Pour the smoothie into two glasses.
5. Serve immediately and enjoy!

Nutritional Values: Calories: 141 Total Fat: 2 g

Saturated Fat: 0 g Cholesterol: 5 mg Sodium: 97 mg
Total Carbohydrate: 26 g Dietary Fiber: 4 g Total Sugars: 18 g Protein: 7 g

Vegan Breakfast Tacos

Preparation time: 15 minutes **Cooking Time:** 15 minutes **Servings:** 4
Ingredients:

- 1 package of extra-firm tofu, drained and crumbled.
- 1 tbsp of olive oil
- 1/2 tsp of garlic powder
- 1/2 tsp of turmeric powder
- Salt and black pepper, to taste
- 4 small whole-grain tortillas
- 1 ripe avocado, sliced.
- 1 small tomato, diced.
- 1/4 cup of chopped fresh cilantro.
- 1 lime, cut into wedges.

Instructions:

1. Heat the olive oil in a large non-stick skillet over medium-high heat.
2. Add the crumbled tofu to the skillet and cook, occasionally stirring, for 5-7 minutes or until lightly browned.
3. Add the garlic powder, turmeric powder, salt, and black pepper to the skillet and stir to combine. Cook for 2-3 minutes or until the tofu is coated and fragrant.
4. Warm the tortillas in a dry skillet or oven for a few minutes until soft and pliable.
5. Divide the tofu scramble between the four tortillas to assemble the vegan breakfast tacos.
6. Top each taco with sliced avocado, diced tomato, and chopped fresh cilantro.
7. Serve each taco with a lime wedge on the side.

Nutritional Values: Calories: 227kcal Total Fat: 13g Saturated Fat: 2g Cholesterol: 0mg Sodium: 224mg Total Carbohydrate: 21g Dietary Fiber: 9g Sugar: 2g Protein: 12g

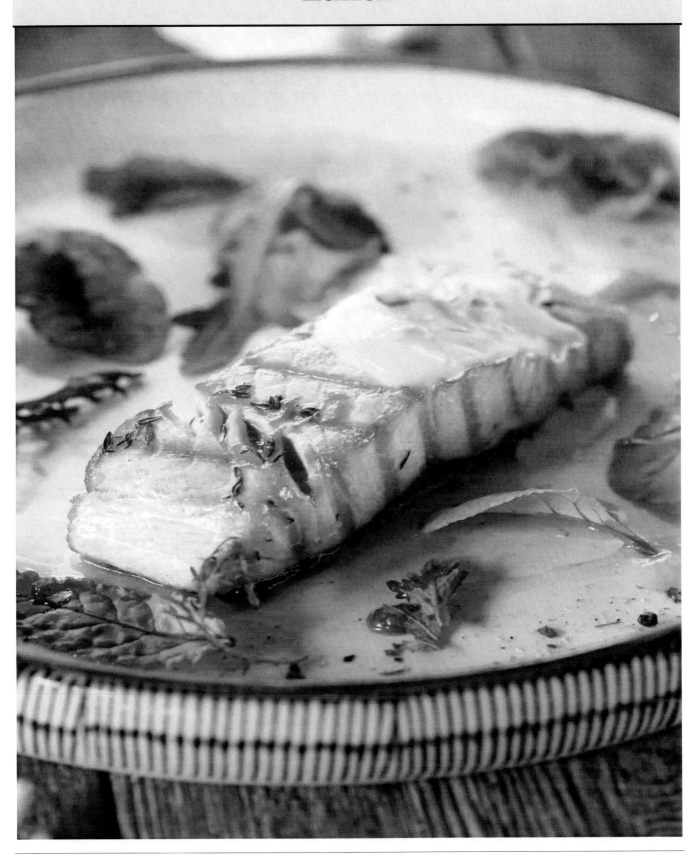

Mediterranean Quinoa Salad

Preparation time: 15 minutes **Cooking Time:** 20 minutes **Servings:** 4

Ingredients:

- 1 cup of uncooked quinoa
- 2 cups of water
- 1/2 cup of chopped fresh parsley.
- 1/2 cup of chopped fresh mint.
- 1/2 cup of crumbled feta cheese
- 1/2 cup of chopped Kalamata olives
- 1/4 cup of chopped red onion.
- 2 tablespoons of extra-virgin olive oil
- 2 tablespoons of red wine vinegar
- Salt and pepper, to taste

Instructions:

1. Rinse the quinoa under cold water.
2. In a medium saucepan, bring the water and quinoa to a boil.
3. Reduce the heat to low and cover the saucepan.
4. Simmer for 15-20 minutes or until the quinoa is tender and the water has been absorbed.
5. In a large mixing bowl, stir the cooked quinoa, chopped fresh parsley, chopped fresh mint, crumbled feta cheese, chopped Kalamata olives, and chopped red onion.
6. Whisk together the extra-virgin olive oil and red wine vinegar in a small mixing bowl.
7. Pour the dressing over the quinoa mixture and toss until well combined.
8. Season with salt and pepper to taste.
9. Serve chilled or at room temperature and enjoy!

Nutritional Values: Calories: 301 Total Fat: 16 g Saturated Fat: 5 g Cholesterol: 22 mg Sodium: 482 mg Total Carbohydrate: 29 g Dietary Fiber: 4 g Total Sugars: 2 g Protein: 10 g

Turkey and Avocado Lettuce Wraps

Preparation time: 15 minutes **Cooking Time:** 0 minutes **Servings:** 4

Ingredients:

- 1 pound of deli-sliced turkey breast
- 2 ripe avocados pitted and sliced.
- 4 large lettuce leaves washed and dried.
- 1/4 cup of low-fat plain Greek yogurt
- 1/4 cup of chopped fresh cilantro.
- 1 tablespoon of lime juice
- Salt and pepper, to taste

Instructions:

1. Lay out the lettuce leaves on a cutting board or work surface.
2. In a mixing bowl, stir the low-fat plain Greek yogurt, chopped fresh cilantro, lime juice, salt, and pepper.
3. Spread the yogurt mixture evenly over each lettuce leaf.
4. Place a few slices of deli-sliced turkey breast and sliced avocado on top of the yogurt mixture.
5. Roll up each lettuce leaf tightly to form a wrap.
6. Serve and enjoy!

Nutritional Values: Calories: 232 Total Fat: 13 g Saturated Fat: 2 g Cholesterol: 42 mg Sodium: 574 mg Total Carbohydrate: 9 g Dietary Fiber: 5 g Total Sugars: 2 g Protein: 21 g

Lentil Soup with Whole-Grain Bread

Preparation time: 10 minutes **Cooking Time:** 40 minutes **Servings:** 6

Ingredients:

- 1 tablespoon of olive oil
- 1 medium onion, chopped.
- 2 cloves of garlic, minced.
- 2 celery stalks, chopped.
- 2 carrots, chopped.
- 1 teaspoon of ground cumin
- 1/2 teaspoon of ground coriander
- 1/2 teaspoon of ground turmeric
- 1/2 teaspoon of paprika
- 1/4 teaspoon of ground cinnamon
- 1/4 teaspoon of cayenne pepper (optional)
- 1 cup of dry brown lentils rinsed and drained.
- 6 cups of low-sodium vegetable broth
- 1 bay leaf

- Salt and pepper, to taste
- 4 slices of whole-grain bread, toasted and cut into cubes.
- Chopped fresh parsley or cilantro for garnish.

Instructions:

1. In a large pot, heat the olive oil over medium heat.
2. Add the chopped onion, minced garlic, celery, and carrots to the pot.
3. Cook for 5-7 minutes or until the vegetables are tender.
4. Add the ground cumin, coriander, turmeric, paprika, ground cinnamon, and cayenne pepper (if used) to the pot.
5. Cook for 1-2 minutes or until fragrant.
6. Add the rinsed and drained brown lentils, low-sodium vegetable broth, and bay leaf to the pot.
7. Bring the soup to a boil, then reduce the heat to low and simmer for 30-35 minutes or until the lentils are tender.
8. Remove the bay leaf from the soup and discard.
9. Season with salt and pepper to taste.
10. Ladle the soup into bowls and top with the toasted whole-grain bread cubes.
11. Garnish with chopped fresh parsley or cilantro, if desired.
12. Serve and enjoy!

Nutritional Values: Calories: 228 Total Fat: 4 g Saturated Fat: 0.5 g Cholesterol: 0 mg Sodium: 198 mg Total Carbohydrate: 36 g Dietary Fiber: 14 g Total Sugars: 4 g Protein: 13 g

Grilled Chicken and Veggie Skewers

Preparation time: 20 minutes **Cooking Time:** 20 minutes **Servings:** 4

Ingredients:

- 1-pound boneless, skinless chicken breasts cut into chunks
- 1 zucchini, sliced into rounds.
- 1 red bell pepper, cut into chunks.
- 1 yellow bell pepper, cut into chunks.
- 1 red onion, cut into chunks.
- 2 tablespoons olive oil
- 2 tablespoons balsamic vinegar
- 1 tablespoon honey
- 1 teaspoon Dijon mustard
- Salt and pepper, to taste
- 1 cup brown rice, cooked according to package directions.

Instructions:

1. Preheat the grill to medium-high heat.
2. Whisk together the olive oil, balsamic vinegar, honey, Dijon mustard, salt, and pepper in a small bowl to make the marinade.
3. Thread the chicken and vegetables onto skewers.
4. Brush the skewers with the marinade, making sure to coat all sides.
5. Grill the skewers for 10-12 minutes, flipping once until the chicken is cooked and the vegetables are tender.
6. Serve the skewers over brown rice.

Nutritional Values: Calories: 374 kcal Total Fat: 10g Saturated Fat: 2g Cholesterol: 65mg Sodium: 144mg Total Carbohydrate: 41g Dietary Fiber: 5g Sugar: 9g Protein: 31g

Roasted Vegetable and Hummus Wrap

Preparation time: 15 minutes **Cooking Time:** 25 minutes **Servings:** 4

Ingredients:

- 1 medium zucchini, sliced.
- 1 red bell pepper, sliced.
- 1 yellow bell pepper, sliced.
- 1 red onion, sliced.
- 2 tablespoons of olive oil
- Salt and pepper, to taste
- 4 large whole-grain tortillas
- 1/2 cup of hummus
- 2 cups of baby spinach leave
- 1/4 cup of crumbled feta cheese

Instructions:

1. Preheat the oven to 425°F (220°C).

2. In a large mixing bowl, toss together the sliced zucchini, red bell pepper, yellow bell pepper, red onion, olive oil, salt, and pepper.
3. Spread the vegetables out in a single layer on a large baking sheet.
4. Roast in the oven for 20-25 minutes or until the vegetables are tender and lightly browned.
5. Lay out the whole-grain tortillas on a work surface.
6. Spread 2 tablespoons of hummus evenly over each tortilla.
7. Top each tortilla with a handful of baby spinach leaves and an equal number of roasted vegetables.
8. Sprinkle the crumbled feta cheese over the vegetables.
9. Roll up each tortilla tightly to form a wrap.
10. Serve and enjoy!

Nutritional Values: Calories: 362 Total Fat: 18 g Saturated Fat: 3 g Cholesterol: 8 mg Sodium: 627 mg Total Carbohydrate: 41 g Dietary Fiber: 10 g Total Sugars: 7 g Protein: 12 g

Tuna and White Bean Salad with Lemon Dressing

Preparation time: 10 minutes **Cooking Time:** none **Servings:** 3
Ingredients:
- 2 cans (5 oz. each) of tuna in water, drained
- 2 cans (15 oz. each) of white beans, rinsed and drained.
- 1 red bell pepper, chopped.
- 1 small red onion thinly sliced.
- 1/4 cup fresh parsley, chopped.
- 1/4 cup fresh lemon juice
- 2 tablespoons extra-virgin olive oil
- 1 clove garlic, minced.
- Salt and pepper to taste

Instructions:
1. Combine the drained tuna, white beans, chopped red bell pepper, thinly sliced red onion, and chopped parsley in a large bowl.

2. In a small bowl, whisk together the fresh lemon juice, extra-virgin olive oil, minced garlic, salt, and pepper until well combined.
3. Pour the lemon dressing over the tuna and white bean mixture and toss until well coated.
4. Serve the salad chilled or at room temperature.

Nutritional Values: Calories: 364 kcal Protein: 28 g Fat: 12 g Carbohydrates: 38 g Fiber: 11 g Sodium: 386 mg

Chickpea and Roasted Vegetable Salad

Preparation time: 15 minutes **Cooking Time:** 25 minutes **Servings:** 4
Ingredients: For the Salad:
- 1 can of chickpeas rinsed and drained.
- 1 red bell pepper, sliced.
- 1 yellow bell pepper, sliced.
- 1 small red onion, sliced.
- 2 cups of baby spinach leave
- 1/4 cup of chopped fresh parsley.
- Salt and pepper, to taste
- 1 tablespoon of olive oil
- For the Dressing:
- 2 tablespoons of balsamic vinegar
- 1 tablespoon of honey
- 1 tablespoon of Dijon mustard
- 1 tablespoon of olive oil
- Salt and pepper, to taste

Instructions:
1. Preheat the oven to 425°F (220°C).
2. In a large mixing bowl, toss the rinsed and drained chickpeas, sliced red bell pepper, sliced yellow bell pepper, sliced red onion, olive oil, salt, and pepper.
3. Spread the vegetables out in a single layer on a large baking sheet.
4. Roast in the oven for 20-25 minutes or until the vegetables are tender and lightly browned.
5. Whisk together the balsamic vinegar, honey, Dijon mustard, olive oil, salt, and pepper in a small mixing bowl to make the dressing.

6. Toss the roasted vegetables, baby spinach leaves, and chopped fresh parsley in a large mixing bowl.

7. Drizzle the balsamic dressing over the salad and toss to combine.

8. Divide the salad evenly among 4 plates.

9. Serve and enjoy!

Nutritional Values: Calories: 192 Total Fat: 7 g Saturated Fat: 1 g Cholesterol: 0 mg Sodium: 192 mg Total Carbohydrate: 29 g Dietary Fiber: 7 g Total Sugars: 12 g Protein: 7 g

Whole-Grain Pasta with Roasted Tomatoes and Spinach

Preparation time: 10 minutes **Cooking Time:** 20 minutes **Servings:** 4

Ingredients:

- 12 ounces of whole-grain pasta
- 2 pints of cherry tomatoes, halved.
- 4 cloves of garlic, minced.
- 2 tablespoons of olive oil
- Salt and pepper, to taste
- 4 cups of baby spinach leave
- 1/4 cup of grated Parmesan cheese

Instructions:

1. Preheat the oven to 400°F (200°C).
2. In a large mixing bowl, toss together the halved cherry tomatoes, minced garlic, olive oil, salt, and pepper.
3. Spread the tomato mixture in a single layer on a large baking sheet.
4. Roast in the oven for 15-20 minutes or until the tomatoes are tender and lightly browned.
5. While the tomatoes are roasting, cook the whole-grain pasta according to the package instructions.
6. Drain the cooked pasta and return it to the pot.
7. Add the roasted tomato mixture and the baby spinach leaves to the pot with the pasta.
8. Toss everything together until the spinach is wilted and the pasta is coated with the tomato juices.

9. Sprinkle the grated Parmesan cheese over the pasta.

10. Serve and enjoy!

Nutritional Values: Calories: 384 Total Fat: 10 g Saturated Fat: 2 g Cholesterol: 5 mg Sodium: 177 mg Total Carbohydrate: 62 g Dietary Fiber: 9 g Total Sugars: 7 g Protein: 14 g

Grilled Salmon with Roasted Vegetables

Preparation time: 10 minutes **Cooking Time:** 20 minutes **Servings:** 4

Ingredients:

- 4 salmon fillets (4-6 oz each), skin removed.
- 1 large zucchini, sliced.
- 1 red bell pepper, sliced.
- 1 yellow bell pepper, sliced.
- 1 small red onion, sliced.
- 2 tablespoons olive oil
- 2 teaspoons dried basil
- Salt and pepper to taste

1. **Instructions:**
2. Preheat the oven to 400°F (200°C).
3. Arrange the sliced zucchini, red and yellow bell peppers, and red onion on a baking sheet lined with parchment paper.
4. Drizzle the vegetables with olive oil and sprinkle with dried basil, salt, and pepper.
5. Toss the vegetables until evenly coated, then spread them out in a single layer on the baking sheet.
6. Roast the vegetables in the oven for 20 minutes or until tender and slightly charred.
7. While the vegetables are roasting, heat a grill pan over medium-high heat.
8. Season the salmon fillets with salt and pepper to taste.
9. Grill the salmon for 4-5 minutes per side or until cooked through.
10. Serve the grilled salmon with the roasted vegetables on the side.

Nutritional Values: Calories: 380 kcal Protein: 34 g Fat: 23 g Carbohydrates: 11 g Fiber: 3 g Sodium: 108 mg

Veggie Burger with Sweet Potato Fries

Preparation time: 30 minutes **Cooking Time:** 30 minutes **Servings:** 4

Ingredients:

- For the Veggie Burger:
- 1 can of black beans rinsed and drained.
- 1/2 cup of cooked brown rice
- 1/4 cup of chopped fresh cilantro.
- 1/4 cup of chopped red onion.
- 2 cloves of garlic, minced.
-
-
- 1 teaspoon of ground cumin
- 1/2 teaspoon of smoked paprika
- Salt and pepper, to taste
- 1 egg
- 1/2 cup of whole-wheat breadcrumbs
- 4 whole-wheat buns
- 4 lettuce leaves
- 4 slices of tomato
- For the Sweet Potato Fries:
- 2 medium sweet potatoes, peeled and cut into thin strips.
- 1 tablespoon of olive oil
- 1/2 teaspoon of smoked paprika
- Salt and pepper, to taste

Instructions:

- Preheat the oven to 400°F (200°C).
- In a large mixing bowl, mash the rinsed and drained black beans with a fork.
- Add the cooked brown rice, chopped cilantro, chopped red onion, minced garlic, ground cumin, smoked paprika, salt, and pepper to the bowl with the mashed black beans.
- Stir everything together until well combined.
- Add the egg and whole-wheat breadcrumbs to the bowl and mix until evenly distributed.
- Form the mixture into 4 patties.
- Place the patties on a lightly oiled baking sheet and bake in the oven for 20-25 minutes or until they are cooked and lightly browned.
- While the veggie burgers are baking, prepare the sweet potato fries.
- Toss the sweet potato strips, olive oil, smoked paprika, salt, and pepper in a large mixing bowl.
- Spread the sweet potato strips in a single layer on a large baking sheet.
- Roast in the preheated oven for 20-25 minutes, or until they are tender and lightly browned.
- Serve the veggie burgers on whole-wheat buns with lettuce leaves, tomato slices, and sweet potato fries on the side.
- Enjoy!

Nutritional Values: Calories: 435 Total Fat: 10 g Saturated Fat: 2 g Cholesterol: 47 mg Sodium: 483 mg Total Carbohydrate: 72 g Dietary Fiber: 17 g Total Sugars: 13 g Protein: 18

Shrimp and Vegetable Stir-Fry with Brown Rice

Preparation time: 15 minutes Cooking **Time:** 20 minutes Servings: 4

Ingredients:

- 1-pound raw shrimp, peeled and deveined
- 3 cups cooked brown rice.
- 1 red bell pepper thinly sliced.
- 1 yellow bell pepper thinly sliced.
- 1 small onion thinly sliced.
- 2 cloves garlic, minced.
- 2 tablespoons olive oil
- 1 tablespoon low-sodium soy sauce
- 1 teaspoon honey
- 1 teaspoon grated ginger
- Salt and pepper to taste

Instructions:

1. Heat a large skillet over medium-high heat. Add 1 tablespoon of olive oil to the skillet.
2. Once the oil is hot, add the shrimp to the skillet and season with salt and pepper. Cook the shrimp for 2-3 minutes on each side or until fully cooked. Remove the shrimp from the skillet and set aside.

3. Add the remaining tablespoon of olive oil to the skillet. Once hot, add the sliced onions, bell peppers, and garlic to the skillet. Cook for 5-7 minutes, stirring occasionally, or until the vegetables are tender.
4. Whisk together the soy sauce, honey, and grated ginger in a small bowl.
5. Add the cooked shrimp back into the skillet with the vegetables. Pour the soy sauce mixture over the shrimp and vegetables and toss everything together until the shrimp and vegetables are coated in the sauce.
6. Serve the shrimp and vegetable stir-fry over cooked brown rice.

Nutritional Values: Calories: 370 kcal Fat: 9g Carbohydrates: 45g Fiber: 6g Protein: 29g Sodium: 260mg

Chicken and Vegetable Stir-Fry

Preparation time: 20 minutes **Cooking Time:** 20 minutes **Servings:** 4
Ingredients:
- 1 cup of brown rice
- 2 cups of water
- 1 tablespoon of olive oil
- 1 pound of boneless, skinless chicken breasts cut into bite-sized pieces.
- 2 cups of sliced mixed vegetables (such as bell peppers, carrots, broccoli, and snap peas)
- 2 cloves of garlic, minced.
- 1 tablespoon of grated fresh ginger
- 2 tablespoons of low-sodium soy sauce
- 1 tablespoon of rice vinegar
- 1 teaspoon of honey
- 1/4 teaspoon of red pepper flakes
- Salt and pepper, to taste

Instructions:
1. In a medium saucepan, bring the water to a boil.
2. Add the brown rice and stir well.
3. Cover the saucepan and reduce the heat to low.
4. Simmer for 45-50 minutes or until the rice is tender and all the water is absorbed.

5. While the rice is cooking, heat the olive oil in a large skillet over medium-high heat.
6. Add the chicken pieces to the skillet and cook for 5-7 minutes or until cooked.
7. Next, add the sliced vegetables, minced garlic, and grated ginger to the skillet.
8. Cook for another 5-7 minutes or until the vegetables are tender-crisp.
9. Whisk together the low-sodium soy sauce, rice vinegar, honey, red pepper flakes, salt, and pepper in a small mixing bowl.
10. Pour the sauce over the chicken and vegetables in the skillet and toss everything together until everything is evenly coated.
11. Serve the chicken and vegetable stir-fry over the cooked brown rice.
12. Enjoy!

Nutritional Values: Calories: 330 Total Fat: 7 g Saturated Fat: 1 g Cholesterol: 65 mg Sodium: 415 mg Total Carbohydrate: 38 g Dietary Fiber: 4 g Total Sugars: 4 g Protein: 29 g

Greek Salad with Chicken and Whole-Grain Pita

Preparation time: 20 minutes **Cooking Time:** 20 minutes **Servings:** 4
Ingredients:
- For the Greek Salad:
- 4 cups of chopped romaine lettuce
- 1 cup of sliced cucumber
- 1 cup of halved cherry tomatoes
- 1/2 cup of sliced red onion
- 1/2 cup of crumbled feta cheese
- 1/4 cup of sliced Kalamata olives
- For the Chicken:
- 1 pound of boneless, skinless chicken breasts
- 2 cloves of garlic, minced.
- 1 tablespoon of dried oregano
- 1 tablespoon of olive oil
- Salt and pepper, to taste
- For the Whole-Grain Pita:
- 4 whole-grain pitas
- 1 tablespoon of olive oil
- 1/4 teaspoon of garlic powder

- Salt and pepper, to taste
- For the Dressing:
- 2 tablespoons of olive oil
- 1 tablespoon of red wine vinegar
- 1/2 teaspoon of dried oregano
- Salt and pepper, to taste

Instructions:

1. Preheat the oven to 400°F (200°C).
2. Combine the chopped romaine lettuce, sliced cucumber, halved cherry tomatoes, red onion, crumbled feta cheese, and sliced Kalamata olives in a large mixing bowl.
3. Toss everything together until well combined.
4. Season the chicken breasts with minced garlic, dried oregano, olive oil, salt, and pepper.
5. Place the chicken on a lightly oiled baking sheet and bake in the preheated oven for 20-25 minutes, until they are cooked through and no longer pink in the center.
6. While the chicken is baking, prepare the whole-grain pita.
7. Whisk together the olive oil, garlic powder, salt, and pepper in a small mixing bowl.
8. Brush the mixture over the surface of the whole-grain pitas.
9. Place the pitas on a baking sheet and bake in the oven for 5-7 minutes or until they are lightly browned and crispy.
10. Whisk together the olive oil, red wine vinegar, dried oregano, salt, and pepper in a small mixing bowl to make the dressing.
11. Once the chicken is done baking, slice it into bite-sized pieces.
12. Divide the Greek salad among four serving plates.
13. Top each salad with the sliced chicken.
14. Drizzle the dressing over the top of the salads.
15. Serve with the whole-grain pitas on the side.
16. Enjoy!

Nutritional Values: Calories: 435 Total Fat: 22 g Saturated Fat: 6 g Cholesterol: 86 mg Sodium: 707 mg Total Carbohydrate: 27 g Dietary Fiber: 5 g Total Sugars: 5 g Protein: 33 g

Black Bean and Vegetable Burrito

Preparation time: 20 minutes **Cooking Time:** 15 minutes **Servings:** 4

Ingredients:

- 1 tablespoon olive oil
- 1 small onion, chopped.
- 2 cloves garlic, minced.
- 1 red bell pepper, chopped.
- 1 zucchini, chopped.
- 1 teaspoon ground cumin
- 1 can (15 ounces) of black beans, rinsed and drained.
- 1/2 cup low-sodium vegetable broth
- 1 tablespoon lime juice
- Salt and black pepper to taste
- 4 whole wheat tortillas (8-inch)
- 1 cup shredded lettuce
- 1/2 cup salsa
- 1/4 cup chopped fresh cilantro.

Instructions:

1. In a large skillet, heat the olive oil over medium heat. Add the onion and garlic and cook for 2-3 minutes until softened.
2. Add the red bell pepper, zucchini, and cumin and cook for another 5-7 minutes until the vegetables are tender.
3. Add the skillet's black beans, vegetable broth, and lime juice. Cook for 2-3 minutes until the liquid is mostly absorbed. Season with salt and black pepper to taste.
4. Warm the tortillas in a microwave or on a skillet over medium heat.
5. To assemble the burritos, place a tortilla on a plate and spoon some black bean mixture onto the center. Top with shredded lettuce, salsa, and cilantro.
6. Fold the bottom edge of the tortilla over the filling, then fold in the sides and roll up tightly.
7. Serve the burritos warm.

Nutritional Values: Calories: 289 kcal Fat: 7.6 g Carbohydrates: 45.4 g Fiber: 11.4 g Protein: 11.4 g Sodium: 345 mg

Grilled Chicken Caesar Salad

Preparation time: 15 minutes **Cooking Time:** 15 minutes **Servings:** 4

Ingredients:

- For the Salad:
- 1-pound boneless, skinless chicken breasts
- 8 cups chopped romaine lettuce.
- 1/2 cup freshly grated Parmesan cheese.
- 1/2 cup whole-grain croutons
- Salt and pepper, to taste
- For the Dressing:
- 1/4 cup plain Greek yogurt.
- 1/4 cup freshly grated Parmesan cheese.
- 2 tablespoons freshly squeezed lemon juice.
- 2 tablespoons extra-virgin olive oil
- 2 cloves garlic, minced.
- Salt and pepper, to taste

Instructions:

1. Preheat a grill or grill pan to medium-high heat.
2. Season the chicken breasts with salt and pepper.
3. Grill the chicken for 5-7 minutes per side or until cooked through and no longer pink in the center.
4. Remove the chicken from the grill and rest for 5 minutes.
5. Meanwhile, prepare the dressing.
6. In a small mixing bowl, whisk together the Greek yogurt, Parmesan cheese, lemon juice, olive oil, minced garlic, salt, and pepper until well combined.
7. Once the chicken has rested, slice it into bite-sized pieces.
8. Combine the chopped romaine lettuce, grated Parmesan cheese, and whole-grain croutons in a large mixing bowl.
9. Toss everything together until well combined.
10. Divide the salad among four serving plates.
11. Top each salad with the sliced chicken.
12. Drizzle the dressing over the top of the salads.
13. Serve immediately and enjoy!

Nutritional Values: Calories: 295 Total Fat: 14 g Saturated Fat: 4 g Cholesterol: 74 mg Sodium: 362 mg Total Carbohydrate: 10 g Dietary Fiber: 3 g Total Sugars: 2 g Protein: 32 g

Tuna Salad with Whole-Grain Crackers

Preparation time: 10 minutes **Cooking Time:** 0 minutes **Servings:** 4

Ingredients:

- 2 cans (5 ounces each) of tuna, drained
- 1/4 cup chopped celery.
- 1/4 cup chopped red onion.
- 1/4 cup chopped bell pepper.
- 2 tablespoons chopped fresh parsley.
- 2 tablespoons lemon juice
- 2 tablespoons extra-virgin olive oil
- Salt and pepper, to taste
- Whole-grain crackers for serving.
- Fresh veggies (such as cucumber slices, carrot sticks, and cherry tomatoes) for serving.

Instructions:

1. Combine the drained tuna, chopped celery, chopped red onion, bell pepper, chopped fresh parsley, lemon juice, extra-virgin olive oil, salt, and pepper in a medium mixing bowl.
2. Mix everything together until well combined.
3. Divide the tuna salad among four serving bowls.
4. Serve the tuna salad with whole-grain crackers and fresh veggies on the side.
5. Enjoy!

Nutritional Values: Calories: 176 Total Fat: 9 g Saturated Fat: 1 g Cholesterol: 23 mg Sodium: 296 mg Total Carbohydrate: 5 g Dietary Fiber: 1 g Total Sugars: 1 g Protein: 19 g

Lentil and Vegetable Soup

Preparation time: 10 minutes **Cooking Time:** 45 minutes **Servings:** 6

Ingredients:

- 1 cup dried green lentils
- 1 tbsp. olive oil
- 1 onion, chopped.
- 3 garlic cloves, minced.
- 2 carrots peeled and chopped.
- 2 celery stalks, chopped.

- 1 zucchini, chopped.
- 4 cups low-sodium vegetable broth
- 1 can (14 oz.) diced tomatoes.
- 1 tsp dried thyme
- 1/2 tsp salt
- 1/4 tsp black pepper
- 6 slices of whole-grain bread

Instructions:

1. Rinse the lentils and drain them. Set aside.
2. Heat the olive oil in a large pot over medium heat. Add the onion and garlic and cook for 3-5 minutes or until the onion is translucent.
3. Add the carrots, celery, and zucchini, and cook for another 5-7 minutes or until the vegetables are tender.
4. Add the lentils, vegetable broth, diced tomatoes, thyme, salt, and black pepper. Bring to a boil, then reduce the heat to low and let simmer for 30-40 minutes or until the lentils are tender.
5. While the soup is simmering, toast the whole-grain bread.
6. Serve the soup hot with a slice of toast on the side.

Nutritional Values: Calories: 238 Fat: 4.5g Saturated Fat: 0.6g Sodium: 410mg Carbohydrates: 37g Fiber: 10g Sugars: 6g Protein: 13g

Chicken and Vegetable Curry

Preparation time: 15 minutes **Cooking Time:** 30 minutes **Servings:** 4

Ingredients:

- 1 tablespoon olive oil
- 1 onion, diced.
- 2 cloves garlic, minced.
- 1 tablespoon grated fresh ginger.
- 2 teaspoons curry powder
- 1/2 teaspoon ground cumin
- 1/4 teaspoon ground turmeric
- 1/4 teaspoon ground cinnamon
- 1/4 teaspoon ground coriander
- 1/4 teaspoon cayenne pepper (optional)
- 2 cups diced cooked chicken breast.

- 2 cups chopped mixed vegetables (such as bell pepper, zucchini, and broccoli)
- 1 can (14.5 ounces) diced tomatoes, undrained.
- 1 cup low-sodium chicken broth
- 1/4 cup chopped fresh cilantro.
- Salt and pepper, to taste
- 2 cups cooked brown rice for serving.

Instructions:

1. Heat the olive oil in a large skillet over medium-high heat.
2. Add the diced onion and cook for 3-4 minutes or until softened.
3. Add the minced garlic and grated ginger and cook for 1-2 minutes or until fragrant.
4. Add the curry powder, ground cumin, ground turmeric, ground cinnamon, ground coriander, and cayenne pepper (if using) to the skillet.
5. Stir everything together until well combined.
6. Add the cooked chicken breast and chopped mixed vegetables to the skillet.
7. Stir everything together until well coated in the spice mixture.
8. Add the diced tomatoes (with their juices) and low-sodium chicken broth to the skillet.
9. Bring the mixture to a boil, then reduce the heat to low and simmer for 15-20 minutes, or until the vegetables are tender and the sauce has thickened.
10. Stir in the chopped fresh cilantro and season with salt and pepper to taste.
11. Serve the chicken and vegetable curry over cooked brown rice.
12. Enjoy!

Nutritional Values: Calories: 365 Total Fat: 8 g Saturated Fat: 1 g Cholesterol: 64 mg Sodium: 396 mg Total Carbohydrate: 44 g Dietary Fiber: 7 g Total Sugars: 8 g Protein: 32 g

Veggie and Hummus Wrap

Preparation time: 10 minutes **Cooking Time:** N/A **Servings:** 1

Ingredients:

- 1 whole wheat tortilla

- 2 tbsp hummus
- 1/4 cup shredded carrots
- 1/4 cup chopped cucumber.
- 1/4 cup sliced bell pepper.
- 1/4 avocado, sliced.
-
- 1/4 cup mixed fresh fruit (such as berries, pineapple, or mango)

Instructions:

1. Lay the whole wheat tortilla flat on a clean surface.
2. Spread 2 tbsp of hummus over the entire tortilla.
3. Place the shredded carrots, chopped cucumber, sliced bell pepper, and sliced avocado in a row down the center of the tortilla.
4. Fold the bottom of the tortilla over the veggies, then fold in the sides.
5. Roll the tortilla up tightly and slice it in half.
6. Serve with a side of mixed fresh fruit.

Nutritional Values: Calories: 313 kcal Fat: 14g Carbohydrates: 43g Fiber: 13g Protein: 8g Sodium: 322mg

Turkey and Veggie Sandwich

Preparation time: 10 minutes **Cooking Time:** 0 minutes **Servings:** 2

Ingredients:

- 4 slices of whole-grain bread
- 4 ounces of sliced turkey breast
- 1/2 avocado, sliced.
- 1/2 cup sliced cucumber.
- 1/2 cup sliced bell pepper.
- 1/4 cup sliced red onion.
- 1/4 cup hummus
- 2 tablespoons Dijon mustard
- Salt and pepper to taste

Instructions:

1. Lay out four slices of whole-grain bread.
2. Spread hummus on two slices of bread and Dijon mustard on the other two slices.
3. Next, layer the sliced turkey, avocado, cucumber, bell pepper, and red onion on the hummus-spread bread slices.
4. Season with salt and pepper to taste.
5. Top with the Dijon mustard-spread bread slices to make two sandwiches.
6. Serve and enjoy!

Nutritional Values: Calories: 350 Total Fat: 12 g Saturated Fat: 2 g Cholesterol: 30 mg Sodium: 550 mg Total Carbohydrate: 43 g Dietary Fiber: 11 g Total Sugars: 7 g Protein: 21 g

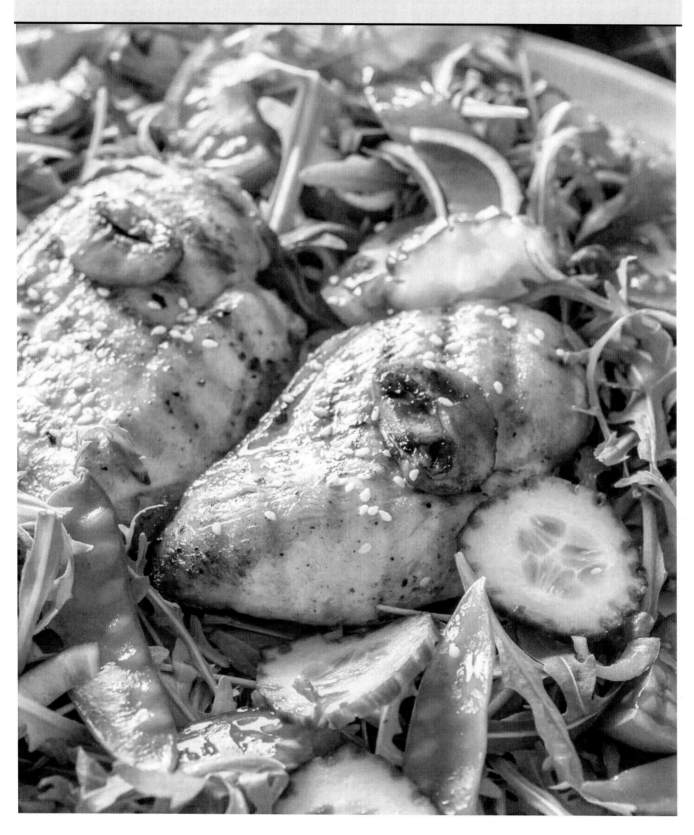

Grilled Chicken and Vegetable Kebabs

Preparation time: 20 minutes **Cooking Time:** 15 minutes **Servings:** 4

Ingredients:

- 1 lb. boneless, skinless chicken breasts, cut into cubes.
- 1 red bell pepper, cut into chunks.
- 1 green bell pepper, cut into chunks.
- 1 zucchini, cut into chunks.
- 1 onion, cut into chunks.
- 1/4 cup olive oil
- 2 cloves garlic, minced.
- 1 tsp dried oregano
- Salt and pepper, to taste
- 2 cups cooked brown rice.
- 4 cups steamed broccoli.

Instructions:

1. Preheat grill to medium-high heat.
2. In a large bowl, combine chicken, bell peppers, zucchini, onion, olive oil, garlic, oregano, salt, and pepper. Toss to coat.
3. Thread chicken and vegetables onto skewers.
4. Grill skewers for 10-15 minutes, or until chicken is cooked through and vegetables are tender.
5. Serve grilled chicken and vegetable kebabs with cooked brown rice and steamed broccoli on the side.

Nutritional Values: Calories: 400 Fat: 16g Carbohydrates: 33g Protein: 35g Sodium: 120mg Fiber: 8g

Vegetable and Lentil Curry

Preparation time: 15 minutes **Cooking Time:** 30 minutes **Servings:** 4

Ingredients:

- 1 cup brown rice
- 2 cups water
- 1 tablespoon olive oil
- 1 onion, chopped.
- 3 garlic cloves, minced.
- 1 tablespoon grated ginger
- 2 teaspoons curry powder
- 1 teaspoon ground turmeric
- 1 teaspoon ground cumin
- 1 teaspoon ground coriander
- 1/2 teaspoon ground cinnamon
- 1/2 teaspoon ground cardamom
- 1/2 teaspoon salt
- 1 red bell pepper, chopped.
- 1 zucchini, chopped.
- 1 can (15 ounces) diced tomatoes.
- 1 can (15 ounces) lentils rinsed and drained.
- 2 cups baby spinach, washed.

Instructions:

1. Rinse the brown rice and add it to a pot with 2 cups of water. Bring to a boil, then reduce the heat to low and cover the pot. Cook for 25-30 minutes or until the rice is tender.
2. Heat the olive oil in a large pan over medium heat. Add the onion, garlic, and ginger and cook for 2-3 minutes until the onion is translucent.
3. Add the curry powder, turmeric, cumin, coriander, cinnamon, cardamom, and salt to the pan and stir to combine.
4. Add the red bell pepper and zucchini to the pan and cook for 5-7 minutes until they are slightly softened.
5. Add the diced tomatoes and lentils to the pan and stir to combine. Cook for 5-7 minutes until the mixture is heated through.
6. Serve the lentil curry over the brown rice with a side of steamed spinach.

Nutritional Values: Calories: 330 kcal Fat: 6 g Carbohydrates: 56 g Fiber: 14 g Protein: 16 g Sodium: 680 mg

Seared Flank Steak

Preparation time: 15 minutes **Cooking Time:** 30 minutes **Servings:** 4

Ingredients:

- 1 lb. flank steak
- 2 medium sweet potatoes peeled and chopped.

- 1 lb. green beans, trimmed.
- 4 cloves garlic, minced.
- 2 sprigs fresh rosemary, chopped.
- 1 tbsp. olive oil
- Salt and black pepper, to taste

Instructions:

1. Preheat the oven to 400°F.
2. In a mixing bowl, combine the sweet potatoes, garlic, rosemary, 1/2 tablespoon of olive oil, and a pinch of salt and black pepper.
3. Spread the sweet potato mixture in a single layer on a baking sheet and bake for 15-20 minutes, or until the sweet potatoes are tender.
4. While the sweet potatoes are cooking, heat a cast-iron skillet over high heat.
5. Rub the flank steak with the remaining olive oil and season it with salt and black pepper.
6. Once the skillet is hot, add the flank steak and cook for 3-4 minutes on each side, or until it's seared and browned on the outside and cooked to your desired level of doneness on the inside.
7. Remove the steak from the skillet and let it rest for a few minutes before slicing it thinly.
8. In the same skillet, add the green beans and cook for 2-3 minutes, or until they're tender but still crisp.
9. Serve the sliced steak with the roasted sweet potatoes and green beans on the side.

Nutritional Values: Calories: 350 kcal Fat: 12 g Carbohydrates: 33 g Fiber: 8 g Protein: 30 g Sodium: 120 mg

Grilled Pork Chops

Preparation time: 20 minutes **Cooking Time:** 35 minutes **Servings:** 4
Ingredients:

- 4 boneless pork chops
- 2 medium sweet potatoes, peeled and cut into 1-inch pieces.
- 1 lb. Brussels sprouts trimmed and halved.
- 1 teaspoon ground cumin
- 1 teaspoon smoked paprika.

- 2 tablespoons olive oil
- Salt and black pepper to taste

Instructions:

1. Preheat the oven to 400°F (200°C).
2. In a large bowl, toss the sweet potatoes and Brussels sprouts with the cumin, paprika, olive oil, salt, and black pepper until evenly coated.
3. Arrange the vegetables in a single layer on a baking sheet and roast for 25 to 30 minutes, until tender and lightly browned, stirring halfway through.
4. While the vegetables are roasting, preheat a grill or grill pan over medium-high heat.
5. Season the pork chops with salt and black pepper to taste. Grill the pork chops for 5 to 6 minutes per side, until cooked through.
6. Serve the grilled pork chops with the roasted sweet potatoes and Brussels sprouts.

Nutritional Values: Calories: 370 kcal Protein: 33 g Fat: 14 g Carbohydrates: 29 g Fiber: 8 g Sodium: 105 mg

Baked Salmon with Mixed Vegetables

Preparation time: 10 minutes **Cooking Time:** 25 minutes **Servings:** 4
Ingredients:

- 4 salmon fillets (4-6 oz. each)
- 2 cups mixed vegetables (such as broccoli, bell peppers, zucchini)
- 2 cloves garlic, minced.
- 1 tsp dried basil
- 1 tsp dried oregano
- 1/4 tsp black pepper
- 1/4 tsp salt
- 2 tbsp. olive oil
- 2 cups cooked quinoa.

Instructions:

1. Preheat the oven to 375°F (190°C).
2. In a bowl, combine the minced garlic, dried basil, dried oregano, black pepper, salt, and olive oil.

3. Place the salmon fillets in a baking dish and rub the garlic mixture over the fillets.
4. Place the mixed vegetables around the salmon fillets in the baking dish.
5. Bake in the preheated oven for 20-25 minutes, until the salmon is cooked through, and the vegetables are tender.
6. Serve the baked salmon and mixed vegetables with a side of cooked quinoa.

Nutritional Values: Calories: 430 kcal Fat: 19 g Saturated Fat: 3 g Sodium: 236 mg Carbohydrates: 24 g Fiber: 4 g Sugar: 2 g Protein: 40 g Potassium: 1132 mg

Lemon and Herb Roasted Chicken

Preparation time: 10 minutes **Cooking Time:** 1-hour **Servings:** 4

Ingredients:

- 4 chicken thighs, skin-on
- 1 lemon juiced and zested.
- 1 tablespoon olive oil
- 2 cloves garlic, minced.
- 1 teaspoon dried thyme
- 1 teaspoon dried rosemary
- Salt and pepper, to taste
- 4 large carrots, peeled and sliced into 1-inch pieces.
- 1 tablespoon honey
- 1 tablespoon balsamic vinegar
- 2 cups cooked brown rice.

Instructions:

1. Preheat the oven to 375°F.
2. In a small bowl, combine the lemon juice, lemon zest, olive oil, garlic, thyme, and rosemary. Mix well.
3. Season the chicken thighs with salt and pepper, then rub the lemon and herb mixture all over the chicken.
4. Place the chicken thighs in a baking dish and roast for 40-45 minutes, until the skin is crispy, and the internal temperature of the chicken reaches 165°F.

5. While the chicken is cooking, prepare the roasted carrots. Toss the sliced carrots with honey, balsamic vinegar, and salt and pepper to taste. Spread the carrots in a single layer on a baking sheet and roast for 25-30 minutes, until tender and lightly caramelized.
6. Serve the roasted chicken with a side of roasted carrots and cooked brown rice.

Nutritional Values: Calories: 395 Fat: 16g Carbohydrates: 34g Fiber: 5g Protein: 29g Sodium: 249mg

Black Bean and Vegetable Quesadillas

Preparation time: 15 minutes **Cooking Time:** 15 minutes **Servings:** 4

Ingredients:

- 1 can of black beans, drained and rinsed.
- 1 red bell pepper, sliced.
- 1 green bell pepper, sliced.
- 1 onion, sliced.
- 1 tbsp. olive oil
- 1 tsp ground cumin
- 1 tsp smoked paprika.
- 4 whole-grain tortillas
- 1/2 cup shredded cheddar cheese
- Salsa, to serve.
- Mixed greens, to serve.

Instructions:

1. Preheat the oven to 350°F (175°C).
2. In a large skillet, heat the olive oil over medium heat. Add the sliced onions and peppers, and sauté for 5-7 minutes until they are tender.
3. Add the black beans, cumin, and smoked paprika to the skillet, and stir until well combined. Cook for another 2-3 minutes until the black beans are heated through.
4. Lay the tortillas on a baking sheet. Divide the black bean and vegetable mixture evenly onto each tortilla, leaving a 1-inch border around the edge.
5. Sprinkle the shredded cheddar cheese over the black bean mixture on each tortilla.

6. Fold the tortillas in half, pressing down lightly.

7. Bake the quesadillas for 8-10 minutes until the cheese is melted and the tortillas are crispy.

8. Serve the quesadillas with salsa and mixed greens on the side.

Nutritional Values: Calories: 340 kcal Fat: 13g Carbohydrates: 42g Fiber: 11g Protein: 16g Sodium: 370mg

Baked Turkey Meatballs

Preparation time: 15 minutes **Cooking Time:** 25 minutes **Servings:** 4
Ingredients:

- For the meatballs:
- 1-pound ground turkey
- 1/2 cup breadcrumbs (preferably whole grain)
- 1 egg
- 1/4 cup chopped fresh parsley.
- 1/4 cup grated Parmesan cheese.
- 1/2 teaspoon garlic powder
- 1/2 teaspoon onion powder
- 1/2 teaspoon salt
- 1/4 teaspoon black pepper
- For the tomato sauce:
- 1 can (28 ounces) crushed tomatoes
- 1 onion, chopped.
- 3 garlic cloves, minced.
- 1 tablespoon olive oil
- 1/2 teaspoon salt
- 1/4 teaspoon black pepper
- 1/4 teaspoon dried oregano
- 1/4 teaspoon dried basil
- For the mixed vegetables:
- 2 cups mixed vegetables
- 1 tablespoon olive oil
- 1/2 teaspoon salt
- 1/4 teaspoon black pepper
- For the whole-grain pasta:
- 8 ounces whole-grain pasta

Instructions:
1. Preheat the oven to 400°F.

2. In a large bowl, combine the ground turkey, breadcrumbs, egg, parsley, Parmesan cheese, garlic powder, onion powder, salt, and black pepper. Mix well.

3. Shape the mixture into 16 meatballs, each about 2 inches in diameter.

4. Place the meatballs on a baking sheet and bake for 15 minutes.

5. Meanwhile, make the tomato sauce. In a large skillet, heat the olive oil over medium heat. Add the onion and garlic and sauté until softened, about 5 minutes.

6. Add the crushed tomatoes, salt, black pepper, oregano, and basil to the skillet. Simmer for 10 minutes.

7. While the meatballs and tomato sauce are cooking, prepare the mixed vegetables. In a large bowl, toss the chopped vegetables with olive oil, salt, and black pepper.

8. Spread the vegetables on a separate baking sheet and roast in the oven for 15 minutes, until tender and lightly browned.

9. Cook the pasta according to package instructions.

10. Serve the meatballs with tomato sauce, mixed vegetables, and whole-grain pasta.

Nutritional Values: Calories: 457 kcal Fat: 16 g Saturated Fat: 4 g Cholesterol: 115 mg Sodium: 1080 mg Carbohydrates: 47 g Fiber: 9 g Sugar: 12 g Protein: 34 g

Beef and Vegetable Stir-Fry

Preparation time: 15 minutes **Cooking Time:** 15 minutes **Servings:** 4
Ingredients:

- 1 lb. beef sirloin thinly sliced.
- 2 tbsp. cornstarch
- 2 tbsp. low-sodium soy sauce
- 2 tbsp. vegetable oil
- 2 cups broccoli florets
- 1 red bell pepper, sliced.
- 1 yellow onion, sliced.
- 2 garlic cloves, minced.
- 1 tsp ginger, minced.

- 1/4 cup beef broth
- Salt and black pepper, to taste
- 2 cups cooked brown rice.

Instructions:

1. In a bowl, mix the beef, cornstarch, and soy sauce. Set aside.
2. Heat 1 tablespoon of vegetable oil in a large skillet over medium-high heat. Add the broccoli and stir-fry for 2-3 minutes until tender. Remove from the skillet and set aside.
3. Add the remaining tablespoon of vegetable oil to the skillet. Add the beef and stir-fry for 3-4 minutes until browned.
4. Add the red bell pepper, onion, garlic, and ginger to the skillet. Stir-fry for another 2-3 minutes until the vegetables are tender.
5. Pour the beef broth into the skillet and bring to a simmer. Stir to scrape any browned bits from the bottom of the skillet. Season with salt and black pepper, to taste.
6. Serve the beef and vegetable stir-fry with cooked brown rice and steamed broccoli on the side.

Nutritional Values: Calories: 420 kcal Fat: 16g Carbohydrates: 34g Fiber: 5g Protein: 35g Sodium: 370mg

Spicy Shrimp and Vegetable Stir-Fry

Preparation time: 10 minutes **Cooking Time:** 15 minutes **Servings:** 4

Ingredients:

- 1-pound large shrimp, peeled and deveined
- 1 red bell pepper, sliced.
- 1 yellow bell pepper, sliced.
- 1 medium onion, sliced.
- 2 cloves garlic, minced.
- 1 tablespoon grated fresh ginger.
- 1 tablespoon low-sodium soy sauce
- 2 teaspoons chili paste.
- 1 teaspoon honey
- 2 tablespoons vegetable oil
- 1 cup brown rice
- 2 cups water

- Salt and black pepper, to taste
- 4 cups fresh spinach leaves washed and dried.

Instructions:

1. Cook brown rice according to package directions.
2. Heat the vegetable oil in a large skillet over medium-high heat. Add the onion and cook until softened, about 2 minutes.
3. Add the garlic and ginger and cook for an additional minute.
4. Add the bell peppers and cook for 2-3 minutes until slightly softened.
5. In a small bowl, whisk together the soy sauce, chili paste, and honey.
6. Add the shrimp to the skillet and cook for 2-3 minutes, until pink and cooked through.
7. Pour the soy sauce mixture over the shrimp and vegetables and toss to coat.
8. Season with salt and black pepper, to taste.
9. Serve the stir-fry over the brown rice with a side of steamed spinach.

Nutritional Values: Calories: 370 kcal Protein: 27g Fat: 10g Carbohydrates: 44g Fiber: 6g Sodium: 385mg

Turkey and Quinoa Stuffed Bell Peppers

Preparation time: 20 minutes **Cooking Time:** 40 minutes **Servings:** 4

Ingredients:

- 4 bell peppers halved and seeded.
- 1-pound ground turkey
- 1 cup cooked quinoa
- 1 small onion, chopped.
- 2 cloves garlic, minced.
- 1 teaspoon dried oregano
- 1 teaspoon dried basil
- 1/2 teaspoon salt
- 1/4 teaspoon black pepper
- 1 cup low-sodium tomato sauce
- 1/4 cup shredded low-fat mozzarella cheese.
- 1/4 cup chopped fresh parsley.
- 1 bunch of asparagus trimmed and steamed.

Instructions:

1. Preheat oven to 375°F.
2. In a large skillet, cook the ground turkey over medium-high heat until browned, stirring frequently to break up the meat.
3. Add the onion and garlic to the skillet and cook until the onion is translucent.
4. Add the cooked quinoa, oregano, basil, salt, and black pepper to the skillet and stir to combine.
5. Add the tomato sauce to the skillet and stir to combine. Cook until the mixture is heated through.
6. Spoon the turkey and quinoa mixture into the bell pepper halves and place them in a baking dish.
7. Cover the baking dish with foil and bake for 25 minutes.
8. Remove the foil from the baking dish, sprinkle the cheese on top of the stuffed peppers, and bake for an additional 10-15 minutes, or until the cheese is melted and the peppers are tender.
9. Serve with steamed asparagus on the side and garnish with chopped parsley.

Nutritional Values: Calories: 290 Fat: 8g Saturated Fat: 2g Cholesterol: 60mg Sodium: 420mg Carbohydrates: 24g Fiber: 6g Sugar: 9g Protein: 29g

Baked Chicken Parmesan

Preparation time: 20 minutes **Cooking Time:** 45 minutes **Servings:** 4

Ingredients:

- 4 boneless, skinless chicken breasts (about 1 1/2 pounds)
- 1/2 cup whole-wheat breadcrumbs
- 1/4 cup grated Parmesan cheese.
- 1 teaspoon dried basil
- 1 teaspoon dried oregano
- 1/2 teaspoon garlic powder
- 1/2 teaspoon onion powder
- 1/4 teaspoon black pepper
- 1 egg, beaten.
- 1 cup tomato sauce
- 4 ounces' part-skim mozzarella cheese, shredded.
- 8 ounces whole-grain pasta
- 2 medium zucchinis, sliced.
- 1 tablespoon olive oil
- Salt and pepper, to taste

Instructions:

1. Preheat the oven to 375°F (190°C).
2. In a shallow dish, combine the breadcrumbs, Parmesan cheese, basil, oregano, garlic powder, onion powder, and black pepper.
3. In another shallow dish, beat the egg.
4. Dip each chicken breast first into the egg, and then into the breadcrumb mixture, coating both sides evenly.
5. Place the chicken breasts in a baking dish coated with cooking spray.
6. Bake for 25-30 minutes, or until the chicken is cooked through and the breadcrumbs are golden brown.
7. While the chicken is baking, cook the whole-grain pasta according to the package directions.
8. In a small saucepan, heat the tomato sauce over low heat.
9. In a separate baking dish, toss the sliced zucchini with olive oil, salt, and pepper.
10. After the chicken has baked for 25-30 minutes, add the shredded mozzarella cheese and tomato sauce on top of each chicken breast.
11. Return the chicken to the oven and bake for another 10-15 minutes, or until the cheese is melted and bubbly.
12. Meanwhile, roast the zucchini in the oven at 375°F (190°C) for 15-20 minutes, or until tender and lightly browned.
13. Serve the chicken with the whole-grain pasta and roasted zucchini on the side.

Nutritional Values: Calories: 522 kcal Fat: 16 g Saturated Fat: 5 g Cholesterol: 160 mg Sodium: 792 mg Carbohydrates: 46 g Fiber: 8 g Sugar: 7 g Protein: 49 g Potassium: 926 mg

Spicy Black Bean and Vegetable Chili

Preparation time: 15 minutes **Cooking Time:** 35 minutes **Servings:** 4

Ingredients:

- 1 tablespoon olive oil
- 1 medium onion, chopped.
- 1 red bell pepper, chopped.
- 1 green bell pepper, chopped.
- 2 cloves garlic, minced.
- 1 teaspoon ground cumin
- 1 teaspoon chili powder
- 1/2 teaspoon smoked paprika.
- 1/2 teaspoon dried oregano
- 1 can (14.5 ounces) diced tomatoes, undrained.
- 1 can (15 ounces) black beans rinsed and drained.
- 1 cup frozen corn kernels
- 1/2 cup water
- 1 tablespoon tomato paste
- Salt and black pepper, to taste
- 2 tablespoons chopped fresh cilantro.

Instructions:

1. Heat olive oil in a large pot over medium heat. Add onion, red and green bell peppers, and garlic. Cook until vegetables are tender, about 5 minutes.
2. Add cumin, chili powder, smoked paprika, and dried oregano. Stir to combine and cook for an additional 2 minutes.
3. Add diced tomatoes, black beans, corn, water, and tomato paste to the pot. Stir to combine and bring to a boil.
4. Reduce heat to low and simmer for 25 minutes, stirring occasionally.
5. Season with salt and black pepper, to taste.
6. Ladle chili into bowls and top with chopped fresh cilantro.

Nutritional Values: Calories: 217kcal Fat: 5g Carbohydrates: 38g Fiber: 11g Protein: 10g Sodium: 537mg

Vegetable and Tofu Kebabs

Preparation time: 15 minutes **Cooking Time:** 20 minutes **Servings:** 4

Ingredients:

- 1 block of firm tofu, pressed and cut into 1-inch cubes.
- 1 red bell pepper, seeded and cut into 1-inch pieces.
- 1 yellow squash, sliced.
- 1 zucchini, sliced.
- 1 red onion, cut into 1-inch pieces.
- 8 cherry tomatoes
- 2 tbsp. olive oil
- 1 tbsp. balsamic vinegar
- 1 tsp dried oregano
- Salt and black pepper to taste
- 2 cups cooked brown rice.
- 4 cups mixed greens

Instructions:

1. Preheat the grill to medium-high heat.
2. In a bowl, whisk together the olive oil, balsamic vinegar, oregano, salt, and black pepper.
3. Thread the tofu, bell pepper, squash, zucchini, red onion, and cherry tomatoes onto skewers.
4. Brush the skewers with the marinade and place them on the grill.
5. Grill for 10-12 minutes, turning occasionally, until the vegetables are tender, and the tofu is lightly browned.
6. Serve the kebabs with brown rice and mixed greens on the side.

Nutritional Values: Calories: 299 kcal Fat: 12g Carbohydrates: 34g Fiber: 6g Protein: 14g Sodium: 71mg

Grilled Sirloin Steak

Preparation time: 10 minutes **Cooking Time:** 25 minutes **Servings:** 5

Ingredients:

- 5 sirloin steaks (4-6 oz. each)
- 1 large red bell pepper, sliced.
- 1 large green bell pepper, sliced.
- 1 medium zucchini, sliced.
- 1 medium yellow squash, sliced.
- 1 small red onion, sliced.
- 2 cloves garlic, minced.
- 1/4 cup olive oil
- 1 tsp dried oregano
- Salt and pepper, to taste
- 1 cup quinoa
- 2 cups water

Instructions:

1. Preheat grill to medium-high heat.
2. In a large bowl, mix sliced bell peppers, zucchini, yellow squash, red onion, minced garlic, olive oil, oregano, salt and pepper.
3. Spread vegetables on a baking sheet and roast in the oven at 375°F for 20-25 minutes or until the vegetables are tender.
4. While the vegetables are roasting, rinse quinoa in a fine mesh strainer and place in a medium saucepan with water. Bring to a boil, then reduce heat and simmer for 15-20 minutes or until the water has been absorbed and the quinoa is tender.
5. Season steaks with salt and pepper and grill for 3-4 minutes per side for medium-rare.
6. Serve the grilled sirloin steak with the roasted mixed vegetables and quinoa on the side.

Nutritional Values: Calories: 465 Fat: 19 g Saturated Fat: 4 g Cholesterol: 80 mg Sodium: 150 mg Carbohydrates: 37 g Fiber: 6 g Sugar: 6 g Protein: 37 g Potassium: 1073 mg Vitamin A: 30% DV Vitamin C: 118% DV Calcium: 7% DV Iron: 30% DV

Roasted Vegetable Lasagne

Preparation time: 30 minutes **Cooking Time:** 1-hour **Servings:** 8

Ingredients:

- 12 whole-grain lasagna noodles
- 2 medium zucchinis, sliced.
- 1 medium eggplant, sliced.
- 1 red bell pepper, sliced.
- 1 yellow bell pepper, sliced.
- 1 large onion, sliced.
- 2 cups baby spinach
- 2 cups marinara sauce
- 1 cup low-fat ricotta cheese
- 1 cup shredded part-skim mozzarella cheese
- 1/4 cup chopped fresh basil.
- 1/4 cup chopped fresh parsley.
- 2 cloves garlic, minced.
- 1 tablespoon olive oil
- Salt and pepper to taste

Instructions:

1. Preheat oven to 375°F (190°C).
2. Cook lasagna noodles according to package instructions. Drain and set aside.
3. Arrange zucchini, eggplant, bell peppers, and onion on a baking sheet. Drizzle with olive oil and sprinkle with garlic, salt, and pepper.
4. Roast vegetables for 20-25 minutes or until they are tender and lightly browned.
5. In a mixing bowl, combine ricotta cheese, spinach, basil, parsley, salt, and pepper.
6. In a 9x13 inch baking dish, spread a layer of marinara sauce on the bottom. Top with a layer of lasagna noodles. Add a layer of roasted vegetables, followed by a layer of the ricotta mixture. Repeat until all ingredients are used up, finishing with a layer of marinara sauce on top.
7. Sprinkle shredded mozzarella cheese over the top layer of marinara sauce.

8. Cover the baking dish with foil and bake for 30 minutes. Remove the foil and bake for an additional 10-15 minutes or until the cheese is melted and bubbly.

9. Remove from oven and let it cool for a few minutes before serving.

Nutritional Values: Calories: 325 Fat: 9g Sodium: 382mg Carbohydrates: 42g Fiber: 10g Sugar: 10g Protein: 19g

Baked Chicken and Vegetable Egg Cups

Preparation time: 15 minutes **Cooking Time:** 25 minutes **Servings:** 6

Ingredients:

- 6 large eggs
- 1/2 cup diced cooked chicken breast.
- 1/4 cup chopped bell pepper.
- 1/4 cup chopped onion.
- 1/4 cup chopped mushrooms.
- 1/4 teaspoon salt
- 1/4 teaspoon black pepper
- 1/4 teaspoon garlic powder
- Cooking spray
- 1 large, sweet potato, peeled and diced.

Instructions:

1. Preheat the oven to 375°F (190°C). Coat a 6-cup muffin tin with cooking spray.

2. In a medium bowl, whisk the eggs, salt, pepper, and garlic powder until well combined.

3. Add the chicken, bell pepper, onion, and mushrooms to the egg mixture and stir to combine.

4. Divide the mixture evenly among the muffin cups.

5. Bake for 20-25 minutes, or until the egg cups are set and golden brown on top.

6. While the egg cups are baking, toss the diced sweet potato with a small amount of cooking spray and place on a baking sheet. Bake for 20-25 minutes or until tender and lightly browned.

7. Serve the egg cups with the roasted sweet potatoes on the side.

Nutritional Values: Calories: 120 kcal Carbohydrates: 8 g Protein: 11 g Fat: 5 g Saturated Fat: 1.5 g Cholesterol: 190 mg Fiber: 1 g Sodium: 220 mg

Lemon and Herb Baked Cod

Preparation time: 10 minutes **Cooking Time:** 20 minutes **Servings:** 4

Ingredients:

- 4 cod fillets (about 6 oz. each)
- 2 tbsp. olive oil
- 2 tbsp. lemon juice
- 2 cloves garlic, minced.
- 1 tsp dried oregano
- 1/2 tsp dried thyme
- Salt and pepper, to taste
- 1 lb. asparagus, trimmed.
- 1 tbsp. balsamic vinegar
- 2 cups cooked brown rice.

Instructions:

1. Preheat oven to 375°F (190°C).

2. In a small bowl, whisk together olive oil, lemon juice, garlic, oregano, thyme, salt, and pepper.

3. Place cod fillets in a baking dish and pour the marinade over them, making sure they are coated evenly.

4. Bake for 15-20 minutes or until the fish is cooked through and flakes easily with a fork.

5. While the fish is baking, toss asparagus with balsamic vinegar and season with salt and pepper. Place on a separate baking sheet and roast for 10-12 minutes or until tender.

6. Serve the baked cod with the roasted asparagus and a side of cooked brown rice.

Nutritional Values: Calories: 337kcal Fat: 10g Carbohydrates: 25g Fiber: 4g Protein: 36g Sodium: 130mg

Chicken and Vegetable Lettuce Wraps

Preparation time: 20 minutes **Cooking Time:** 15 minutes **Servings:** 4

Ingredients:

- 1-pound boneless, skinless chicken breast, cut into small pieces
- 2 tablespoons olive oil
- 1 red bell pepper, chopped.
- 1 yellow bell pepper, chopped.
- 1 small onion, chopped.
- 2 cloves garlic, minced.
- 1 teaspoon ground ginger
- 1/4 teaspoon red pepper flakes
- 1/4 cup low-sodium soy sauce
- 1/4 cup natural peanut butter
- 2 tablespoons honey
- 2 tablespoons rice vinegar
- 1 tablespoon sesame oil
- 1 head of iceberg lettuce washed and leaves separated.
- 1 cup shelled edamame, steamed.

Instructions:

1. In a large skillet, heat the olive oil over medium-high heat. Add the chicken and cook for 5-7 minutes, or until no longer pink.
2. Add the bell peppers, onion, garlic, ginger, and red pepper flakes to the skillet. Cook for an additional 5-7 minutes, or until the vegetables are tender.
3. In a small bowl, whisk together the soy sauce, peanut butter, honey, rice vinegar, and sesame oil.
4. Pour the sauce over the chicken and vegetables in the skillet. Stir to combine and cook for an additional 2-3 minutes, or until the sauce has thickened slightly.
5. To serve, spoon the chicken and vegetable mixture onto individual lettuce leaves. Drizzle with additional sauce, if desired. Serve with steamed edamame on the side.

Nutritional Values: Calories: 417kcal Fat: 19g Carbohydrates: 26g Fiber: 5g Protein: 36g Sodium: 536mg

Mushroom and Spinach Stuffed Pork Tenderloin

Preparation time: 30 minutes **Cooking Time:** 45 minutes **Servings:** 4

Ingredients:

- 1 pork tenderloin (about 1 pound)
- 1 cup chopped mushrooms.
- 2 cups fresh spinach
- 2 cloves garlic, minced.
- 1/4 cup grated Parmesan cheese.
- 1 teaspoon dried thyme
- 1/4 teaspoon salt
- 1/4 teaspoon black pepper
- 2 cups diced root vegetables (carrots, parsnips, turnips)
- 2 tablespoons olive oil

Instructions:

1. Preheat oven to 375°F (190°C).
2. Using a sharp knife, make a lengthwise cut down the center of the pork tenderloin, but not all the way through. Open the tenderloin up like a book and lay it flat.
3. In a skillet, cook mushrooms and garlic until tender. Add spinach and cook until wilted.
4. Stir in Parmesan cheese, thyme, salt, and black pepper.
5. Spread the mushroom and spinach mixture over the opened pork tenderloin.
6. Roll the tenderloin up tightly and tie it with kitchen twine.
7. Place the pork tenderloin in a baking dish and roast for 30-35 minutes or until the internal temperature reaches 145°F (63°C).
8. While the pork tenderloin is cooking, toss the diced root vegetables in olive oil and spread them in a single layer on a baking sheet.
9. Roast the vegetables in the oven for 20-25 minutes or until tender and lightly browned.
10. Serve the stuffed pork tenderloin sliced with the roasted root vegetables on the side.

Nutritional Values: Calories: 343 Fat: 16g Saturated Fat: 4g Cholesterol: 95mg Sodium: 262mg Carbohydrates: 15g Fiber: 3g Sugar: 5g Protein: 35g

Main Recipes

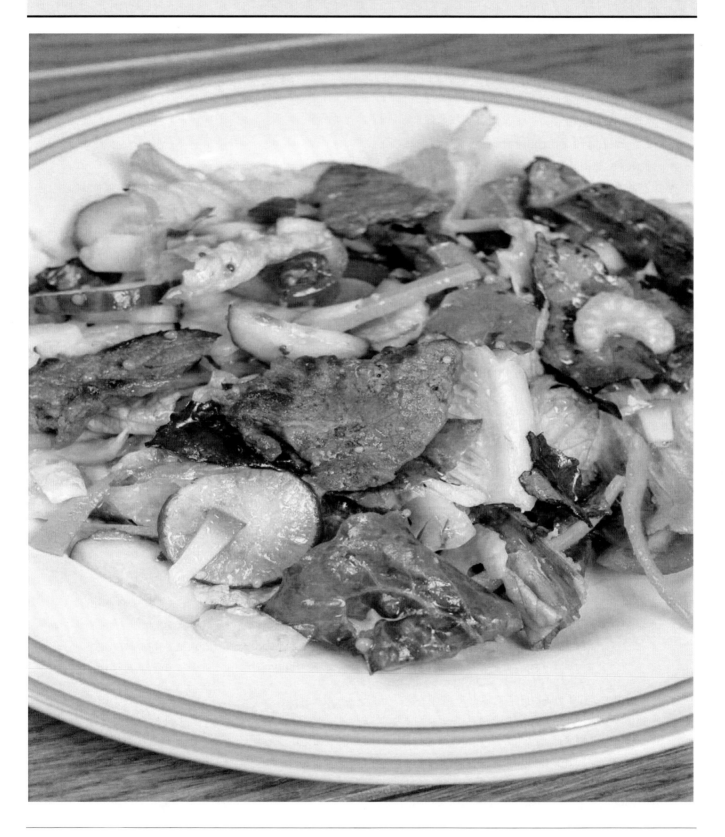

Grilled Salmon with Quinoa

Preparation time: 10 minutes **Cooking Time:** 20 minutes **Servings:** 4

Ingredients:

- 4 salmon fillets, skin removed.
- 1 cup quinoa
- 2 cups low-sodium vegetable broth
- 1 red bell pepper, diced.
- 1 yellow bell pepper, diced.
- 1 small red onion, diced.
- 2 cloves garlic, minced.
- 2 tbsp olive oil
- Salt and pepper, to taste
- Lemon wedges for serving.

Instructions:

1. Preheat the grill to medium-high heat.
2. Rinse quinoa in a fine-mesh strainer and transfer to a medium saucepan with vegetable broth. Bring to a boil over high heat. Reduce heat to low, cover, and simmer for 15-20 minutes or until the quinoa is cooked and the liquid is absorbed.
3. While the quinoa is cooking, prepare the vegetables by mixing the bell peppers, red onion, garlic, olive oil, salt, and pepper in a large bowl.
4. Cut 4 pieces of aluminum foil, about 12x12 inches each. Divide the vegetable mixture evenly among the 4 foil pieces, placing it in the center of each piece.
5. Place a salmon fillet on top of the vegetables in each foil piece. Season the salmon with salt and pepper.
6. Fold the foil to make a packet, allowing steam to circulate. Seal the edges well.
7. Grill the packets for 10-12 minutes until the salmon is cooked and flakes easily with a fork.
8. Serve the salmon on a bed of cooked quinoa with mixed vegetables. Squeeze lemon wedges over the salmon, if desired.

Nutritional Values: Calories: 429 Fat: 18g Carbohydrates: 32g Fiber: 5g Protein: 36g Sodium: 198mg

Vegetable and Lentil Curry

Preparation time: 15 minutes **Cooking Time:** 45 minutes **Servings:** 4

Ingredients:

- 1 cup brown rice
- 1 tablespoon olive oil
- 1 onion, chopped.
- 3 cloves garlic, minced.
- 1 tablespoon grated ginger
- 2 tablespoons curry powder
- 1 teaspoon ground cumin
- 1 teaspoon ground coriander
- 1 teaspoon turmeric
- 1 can (15 oz.) diced tomatoes, undrained.
- 1 can (15 oz.) lentils, drained and rinsed.
- 1 sweet potato peeled and diced.
- 2 cups chopped fresh spinach.
- Salt and pepper, to taste

Instructions:

1. Cook brown rice according to package instructions.
2. In a large skillet, heat olive oil over medium heat. Add onion and cook for 5 minutes or until softened.
3. Add garlic, ginger, curry powder, cumin, coriander, and turmeric to the skillet. Cook for 1-2 minutes or until fragrant.
4. Add diced tomatoes, lentils, and sweet potato to the skillet. Bring to a boil, then reduce heat to low and let simmer for 20-25 minutes or until the sweet potato is cooked.
5. Stir in chopped spinach and cook for 1-2 minutes or until wilted.
6. Season with salt and pepper to taste.
7. Serve the lentil curry over cooked brown rice.

Nutritional Values: Calories: 322 kcal Fat: 5 g Carbohydrates: 58 g Fiber: 14 g Protein: 14 g Sodium: 360 mg

Lemon and Herb Roasted Chicken

Preparation time: 15 minutes **Cooking Time:** 1 hour 30 minutes **Servings:** 4

Ingredients:

- 4 chicken breasts, skin on
- 1 lemon, sliced.
- 2 garlic cloves, minced.
- 2 tbsp olive oil
- 1 tbsp dried thyme
- 1 tbsp dried rosemary
- Salt and black pepper to taste
- 4 sweet potatoes peeled and cubed.
- 1/2 cup unsweetened almond milk
- 1 tbsp ghee

Instructions:

1. Preheat oven to 375°F.
2. Mix minced garlic, olive oil, dried thyme, dried rosemary, salt, and black pepper in a small bowl.
3. Place the chicken breasts in a roasting pan and rub the garlic and herb mixture over them.
4. Add sliced lemon on top of the chicken breasts.
5. Roast in the preheated oven for 1 hour and 15 minutes or until the internal temperature of the chicken reaches 165°F.
6. While the chicken is cooking, prepare the sweet potato mash. Boil sweet potato cubes in salted water until soft and easily mashed.
7. Drain the sweet potatoes and add them back to the pot.
8. Add almond milk and ghee and mash the sweet potatoes until smooth.
9. Season with salt and black pepper to taste.
10. Serve the roasted chicken with a side of sweet potato mash.

Nutritional Values: Calories: 421 kcal Fat: 14 g Carbohydrates: 33 g Fiber: 6 g Protein: 42 g Sodium: 191 mg

Grilled Shrimp Skewers

Preparation time: 15 minutes **Cooking Time:** 10 minutes **Servings:** 4

Ingredients:

- 1 lb. large shrimp peeled and deveined.
- 1 red bell pepper, cut into chunks.
- 1 green bell pepper, cut into chunks.
- 1 yellow squash, sliced into rounds.
- 1 zucchini, sliced into rounds.
- 1 red onion, cut into chunks.
- 1/4 cup olive oil
- 2 tbsp lemon juice
- 1 tsp dried oregano
- 1/2 tsp garlic powder
- Salt and pepper, to taste

Instructions:

1. Preheat the grill to medium-high heat.
2. Whisk together olive oil, lemon juice, oregano, garlic powder, salt, and pepper in a small bowl.
3. Thread shrimp and vegetables onto skewers, alternating as desired.
4. Brush skewers with the olive oil mixture.
5. Place skewers on the grill and cook for 3-4 minutes per side or until shrimp is pink and cooked through and vegetables are tender.
6. Serve hot with a side of mixed greens.

Nutritional Values: Calories: 250kcal Carbohydrates: 10g Protein: 22g Fat: 14g Saturated Fat: 2g Cholesterol: 168mg Sodium: 270mg Potassium: 483mg Fiber: 3g Sugar: 5g Vitamin A: 1982IU Vitamin C: 77mg Calcium: 113mg Iron: 3mg

Turkey and Quinoa Stuffed Bell Peppers

Preparation time: 20 minutes **Cooking Time:** 45 minutes **Servings:** 4

Ingredients:

- 4 bell peppers (any color)
- 1-pound ground turkey
- 1/2 cup quinoa
- 1 onion, chopped.

- 2 cloves garlic, minced.
- 1 teaspoon ground cumin
- 1 teaspoon smoked paprika.
- 1/2 teaspoon salt
- 1/4 teaspoon black pepper
- 1 can (14.5 oz.) diced tomatoes, drained.
- 1/2 cup low-sodium chicken broth
- 1/4 cup chopped fresh parsley.

Instructions:

1. Preheat the oven to 375°F.
2. Cut off the tops of the bell peppers and remove the seeds and membranes. Place the bell peppers in a baking dish and set aside.
3. Over medium heat, cook the ground turkey in a large skillet until browned and cooked through, about 5-7 minutes. Drain any excess fat.
4. Add the quinoa, onion, garlic, cumin, smoked paprika, salt, and black pepper to the skillet. Cook for 5 minutes or until the onion is soft.
5. Add the diced tomatoes and chicken broth to the skillet and bring to a simmer. Cook for 5 minutes or until the liquid is mostly absorbed.
6. Remove the skillet from heat and stir in the chopped parsley.
7. Spoon the turkey-quinoa mixture into the bell peppers, filling them to the top.
8. Cover the baking dish with foil and bake for 30 minutes.
9. Remove the foil and bake for 10-15 minutes until the peppers are tender and the filling is hot and bubbly.

Nutritional Values: Calories: 255 kcal Fat: 7 g Carbohydrates: 22 g Fiber: 5 g Protein: 28 g Sodium: 409 mg

Baked Salmon with Roasted Asparagus

Preparation time: 15 minutes **Cooking Time:** 25 minutes **Servings:** 4
Ingredients:

- 4 salmon fillets, skin removed.
- 1 lb. asparagus, trimmed.

- 2 medium sweet potatoes, peeled and cut into fries.
- 2 tbsp. olive oil
- 1 tsp garlic powder
- 1 tsp dried thyme
- 1/2 tsp salt
- 1/4 tsp black pepper

Instructions:

1. Preheat the oven to 400°F (200°C). Line two baking sheets with parchment paper.
2. Mix the garlic powder, thyme, salt, and black pepper in a small bowl.
3. Place the salmon fillets on one of the prepared baking sheets. Sprinkle the spice mixture evenly over the salmon.
4. Toss the asparagus with 1 tablespoon of olive oil in a large bowl. Spread them out on the other prepared baking sheet.
5. Toss the sweet potato fries in the same bowl with the remaining tablespoon of olive oil. Arrange them in a single layer on the same baking sheet as the asparagus.
6. Place both baking sheets in the oven and bake for 20-25 minutes until the salmon is cooked and the sweet potato fries are crispy.
7. Serve the baked salmon with roasted asparagus and sweet potato fries on the side.

Nutritional Values: Calories: 420 kcal Protein: 32g Carbohydrates: 28g Fat: 20g Saturated Fat: 3g Cholesterol: 78mg Fiber: 6g Sodium: 414mg

Spinach and Feta Stuffed Chicken Breasts

Preparation time: 15 minutes **Cooking Time:** 30 minutes **Servings:** 4
Ingredients:

- 4 boneless, skinless chicken breasts
- 1/2 cup crumbled feta cheese
- 1/2 cup chopped fresh spinach.
- 1/4 cup chopped sun-dried tomatoes.
- 2 cloves garlic, minced.
- 1 tablespoon olive oil
- Salt and pepper to taste

- 2 cups chopped mixed vegetables (such as zucchini, bell peppers, and onions)
- 1 tablespoon balsamic vinegar

Instructions:

1. Preheat the oven to 375°F (190°C).
2. Mix the feta cheese, spinach, sun-dried tomatoes, and garlic in a small bowl.
3. Cut a pocket into the side of each chicken breast using a sharp knife. Stuff each chicken breast with the spinach and feta mixture.
4. Brush the chicken breasts with olive oil and season with salt and pepper.
5. Place the stuffed chicken breasts on a baking sheet and bake for 25-30 minutes, until cooked through and no longer pink in the center.
6. While the chicken is cooking, toss the chopped vegetables with olive oil and balsamic vinegar. Spread them on a separate baking sheet and roast for 15-20 minutes until tender and slightly caramelized.
7. Serve the stuffed chicken breasts with roasted vegetables.

Nutritional Values: Calories: 272 Fat: 10g Carbohydrates: 8g Fiber: 3g Protein: 36g Sodium: 302mg

Beef and Vegetable Stir-Fry

Preparation time: 15 minutes **Cooking Time:** 20 minutes **Servings:** 4

Ingredients:

- 1-pound flank steak thinly sliced.
- 2 tablespoons low-sodium soy sauce
- 1 tablespoon cornstarch
- 1 tablespoon sesame oil
- 1 red bell pepper, sliced.
- 1 green bell pepper, sliced.
- 1 small onion, sliced.
- 1 cup broccoli florets
- 1 tablespoon grated ginger
- 2 cloves garlic, minced.
- 1/4 teaspoon red pepper flakes (optional)
- 3 cups cooked brown rice.

Instructions:

1. In a medium bowl, whisk together the soy sauce and cornstarch. Add the sliced beef and stir to coat.
2. Heat the sesame oil in a large skillet or wok over high heat. Add the beef and stir-fry for 2-3 minutes until browned. Remove the meat from the skillet and set aside.
3. Add bell peppers, onion, and broccoli in the same skillet. Stir-fry for 3-4 minutes until the vegetables are tender-crisp.
4. Add the ginger, garlic, and red pepper flakes (if using) to the skillet and stir-fry for an additional minute.
5. Return the beef to the skillet and stir to combine with the vegetables.
6. Serve the stir-fry over cooked brown rice.

Nutritional Values: Calories: 353 kcal Fat: 9 g Saturated Fat: 2 g Carbohydrates: 37 g Fiber: 5 g Protein: 30 g Sodium: 439 mg

Grilled Pork Chops with Roasted Brussels Sprouts

Preparation time: 15 minutes **Cooking Time:** 40 minutes **Servings:** 4

Ingredients:

- 4 bone-in pork chops
- 1/4 cup balsamic vinegar
- 1/4 cup olive oil
- 2 garlic cloves, minced.
- 1 teaspoon dried thyme
- Salt and black pepper, to taste
- 1 pound Brussels sprouts trimmed and halved.
- 2 medium sweet potatoes peeled and cubed.

Instructions:

1. Preheat oven to 400°F (200°C).
2. Whisk together balsamic vinegar, olive oil, garlic, thyme, salt, and black pepper in a small bowl.
3. Place the pork chops in a large resalable bag and pour the marinade over them. Seal the bag and toss it to coat evenly. Marinate in the refrigerator for at least 30 minutes.

4. Toss the Brussels sprouts and sweet potatoes with olive oil, salt, and black pepper in a large bowl. Arrange them in a single layer on a baking sheet.

5. Roast the vegetables for 25-30 minutes, stirring once halfway through, until they are tender and browned.

6. Preheat a grill to medium-high heat. Grill the pork chops for 4-5 minutes per side until they reach an internal temperature of 145°F (63°C).

7. Let the pork chops rest for 5 minutes before serving with the roasted Brussels sprouts and sweet potatoes.

Nutritional Values: Calories: 420kcal Fat: 20g Saturated Fat: 4g Cholesterol: 75mg Sodium: 195mg Carbohydrates: 29g Fiber: 7g Sugar: 7g Protein: 31g

Spicy Black Bean and Vegetable Quesadillas

Preparation time: 10 minutes **Cooking Time:** 20 minutes **Servings:** 4

Ingredients:

- 1 can black beans, drained and rinsed.
- 1 red bell pepper, chopped.
- 1 small onion, chopped.
- 2 cloves garlic, minced.
- 1 teaspoon cumin
- 1 teaspoon chili powder
- 4 whole-grain tortillas
- 1 cup shredded reduced-fat cheddar cheese.
- 1/4 cup chopped fresh cilantro.
- Salsa, for serving.

Instructions:

1. Preheat the oven to 350°F.

2. In a large skillet over medium heat, sauté the bell pepper, onion, and garlic until the vegetables are tender, about 5 minutes.

3. Add the black beans, cumin, and chili powder to the skillet and stir until well combined. Cook for an additional 2-3 minutes.

4. Place a tortilla on a baking sheet and sprinkle with 1/4 cup of shredded cheese. Spoon 1/4 of the black bean mixture onto one half of the tortilla, then fold the other half over to create a half-moon shape.

5. Repeat with the remaining tortillas, cheese, and black bean mixture.

6. Bake the quesadillas for 10-12 minutes or until the cheese is melted and the tortillas are lightly browned.

7. Sprinkle the cilantro over the quesadillas and serve with salsa on the side.

Nutritional Values: Calories: 315 kcal Fat: 9 g Saturated Fat: 4 g Sodium: 524 mg Carbohydrates: 44 g Fiber: 12 g Sugar: 4 g Protein: 16 g

Sides

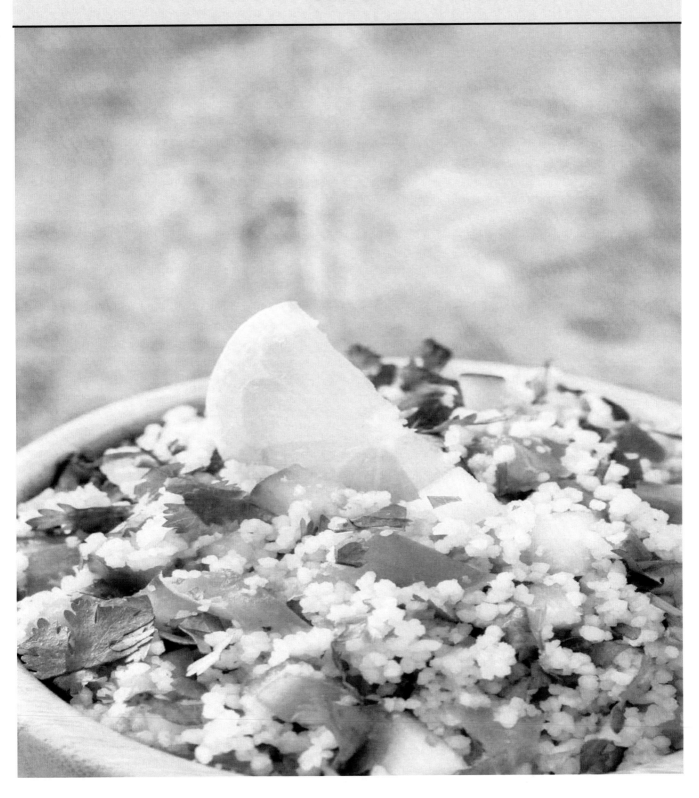

Steamed Green Beans

Preparation time: 10 minutes **Cooking Time:** 10 minutes **Servings:** 4

Ingredients:

- 1 lb. fresh green beans, ends trimmed.
- 2 tbsp. sliced almonds.
- 1 tbsp. extra-virgin olive oil
- 1 garlic clove, minced.
- 1 tbsp. fresh lemon juice
- Salt and pepper to taste

Instructions:

1. Fill a large pot with 1-2 inches of water and bring to a boil over high heat.
2. Place the green beans in a steamer basket or colander and place it over the pot of boiling water. Cover the pot with a lid and steam the green beans for 5-8 minutes, or until tender but still slightly crisp.
3. While the green beans are steaming, heat a small skillet over medium heat. Add the sliced almonds and toast them for 2-3 minutes, or until lightly browned and fragrant. Remove from heat and set aside.
4. In a small bowl, whisk together the olive oil, minced garlic, and lemon juice.
5. Once the green beans are cooked, transfer them to a serving dish and drizzle with the lemon-garlic dressing. Season with salt and pepper to taste.
6. Sprinkle the toasted almonds over the top of the green beans.
7. Serve immediately.

Nutritional Values: Calories: 80 Fat: 5g Carbohydrates: 9g Protein: 3g Fiber: 4g Sodium: 5mg

Roasted Brussels Sprouts with Balsamic Glaze

Preparation time: 10 minutes **Cooking Time:** 25 minutes **Servings:** 4

Ingredients:

- 1 lb. Brussels sprouts trimmed and halved.
- 2 tbsp. olive oil

- Salt and pepper, to taste
- 1/4 cup balsamic vinegar
- 1 tbsp. honey

Instructions:

1. Preheat the oven to 400°F (200°C).
2. In a large bowl, toss the Brussels sprouts with olive oil, salt, and pepper until well coated.
3. Spread the Brussels sprouts out in a single layer on a baking sheet.
4. Roast the Brussels sprouts in the oven for 20-25 minutes, until they are tender and lightly browned.
5. While the Brussels sprouts are roasting, prepare the balsamic glaze. In a small saucepan, combine the balsamic vinegar and honey. Bring to a boil over medium heat, then reduce the heat and simmer until the mixture has thickened and reduced by about half.
6. Drizzle the balsamic glaze over the roasted Brussels sprouts and toss to coat.
7. Serve immediately.

Nutritional Values: Calories: 104kcal Fat: 7g Saturated Fat: 1g Cholesterol: 0mg Sodium: 21mg Potassium: 329mg Carbohydrates: 10g Fiber: 2g Sugar: 6g Protein: 2g Vitamin A: 11% Vitamin C: 96% Calcium: 3% Iron: 6%

Roasted Sweet Potato Wedges

Preparation time: 15 minutes **Cooking Time:** 30 minutes **Servings:** 6

Ingredients:

- 3 large, sweet potatoes, cut into wedges.
- 2 cloves garlic, minced.
- 1 tablespoon fresh thyme leaves
- 1 tablespoon olive oil
- 1/4 teaspoon salt
- 1/4 teaspoon black pepper

Instructions:

1. Preheat the oven to 400°F (200°C).
2. In a large bowl, combine the sweet potato wedges, minced garlic, thyme leaves, olive oil, salt, and black pepper. Toss to coat the sweet potato wedges evenly.
3. Arrange the sweet potato wedges in a single layer on a baking sheet.

4. Roast the sweet potato wedges in the preheated oven for 25-30 minutes, or until they are tender and lightly browned on the outside.
5. Serve the sweet potato wedges hot.

Nutritional Values: Calories: 127 Fat: 4.5g Saturated Fat: 0.6g Sodium: 176mg Carbohydrates: 21.4g Fiber: 3.3g Sugar: 6.4g Protein: 1.8g

Grilled Asparagus with Lemon and Parmesan

Preparation time: 5 minutes **Cooking Time:** 10 minutes **Servings:** 4

Ingredients:
- 1-pound asparagus, ends trimmed.
- 1 tablespoon olive oil
- 1 lemon zested and juiced.
- 1/4 cup grated parmesan cheese.
- Salt and pepper to taste

Instructions:
1. Preheat grill to medium-high heat.
2. In a large bowl, toss asparagus with olive oil, lemon zest, salt, and pepper.
3. Grill asparagus for 5-7 minutes, turning occasionally, until tender and lightly charred.
4. Remove asparagus from the grill and place on a serving dish.
5. Drizzle lemon juice over the asparagus and sprinkle with parmesan cheese.
6. Serve immediately.

Nutritional Values: Calories: 70 Fat: 5g Protein: 4g Carbohydrates: 5g Fiber: 2g Sodium: 90mg

Steamed or Roasted Broccoli

Preparation time: 5 minutes **Cooking Time:** 15-20 minutes **Servings:** 4

Ingredients:
- 1 head of broccoli, chopped into florets.
- 2 cloves of garlic, minced.
- 1 lemon zested and juiced.
- 2 tablespoons of olive oil
- Salt and pepper to taste

Instructions:

1. Preheat your oven to 400°F (200°C) if roasting the broccoli or fill a pot with an inch of water and bring it to a boil if steaming the broccoli.
2. In a mixing bowl, whisk together the olive oil, minced garlic, lemon zest, lemon juice, salt, and pepper.
3. Add the broccoli florets to the mixing bowl and toss them until they are evenly coated in the seasoning mixture.
4. If roasting the broccoli, spread the florets out onto a baking sheet and roast them for 15-20 minutes until they are tender and slightly browned.
5. If steaming the broccoli, place the florets into a steamer basket and cover the pot with a lid. Steam the broccoli for 5-7 minutes until they are tender but still slightly crisp.
6. Serve the steamed or roasted broccoli hot as a side dish.

Nutritional Values: Calories: 82 kcal Fat: 7 g Carbohydrates: 5 g Fiber: 2 g Protein: 2 g Sodium: 31 mg

Mixed Vegetable and Quinoa Salad

Preparation time: 15 minutes **Cooking Time:** 25 minutes **Servings:** 4

Ingredients:
- 1 cup uncooked quinoa
- 2 cups water
- 1 red bell pepper, diced.
- 1 yellow bell pepper, diced.
- 1 cup cherry tomatoes, halved.
- 1/2 red onion, diced.
- 1/4 cup chopped fresh parsley.
- 1/4 cup chopped fresh mint.
- 2 tbsp extra-virgin olive oil
- 2 tbsp lemon juice
- 1 clove garlic, minced.
- Salt and black pepper, to taste

Instructions:
1. Rinse quinoa in a fine mesh strainer and place in a medium saucepan with water. Bring to a boil over medium-high heat, then reduce heat

to low, cover, and simmer for 15-20 minutes until quinoa is tender and water is absorbed.

2. In a large mixing bowl, combine cooked quinoa, red and yellow bell peppers, cherry tomatoes, red onion, parsley, and mint.

3. In a small bowl, whisk together olive oil, lemon juice, garlic, salt, and black pepper to make the vinaigrette.

4. Pour the vinaigrette over the quinoa and vegetable mixture and toss to combine.

5. Serve the salad immediately, or chill in the refrigerator for at least an hour before serving.

Nutritional Values: Calories: 235 kcal Fat: 9.2 g Protein: 7.1 g Carbohydrates: 33.7 g Fiber: 5.1 g Sodium: 93 mg

Roasted Garlic and Herb Roasted Potatoes

Preparation time: 10 minutes **Cooking Time:** 30-40 minutes **Servings:** 4
Ingredients:

- 1 lb. baby potatoes, halved.
- 1 tbsp. olive oil
- 2 cloves garlic, minced.
- 1 tsp. dried rosemary
- 1 tsp. dried thyme
- Salt and pepper, to taste

Instructions:

1. Preheat oven to 400°F (200°C).
2. In a large bowl, mix the halved potatoes, olive oil, minced garlic, rosemary, thyme, salt, and pepper.
3. Spread the potato mixture in a single layer on a baking sheet.
4. Roast the potatoes for 30-40 minutes or until they are tender and crispy on the outside.
5. Serve immediately.

Nutritional Values: Calories: 120 kcal Fat: 4 g Carbohydrates: 20 g Fiber: 2 g Protein: 2 g Sodium: 80 mg

Steamed or Roasted Carrots with Honey

Preparation time: 10 minutes **Cooking Time:** 25 minutes **Servings:** 4
Ingredients:

- 1-pound carrots, peeled and sliced
- 2 tablespoons olive oil
- 1 tablespoon honey
- 1 teaspoon dried thyme
- Salt and pepper to taste

Instructions:

1. Preheat oven to 400°F (200°C).
2. In a large bowl, whisk together olive oil, honey, thyme, salt, and pepper.
3. Add sliced carrots to the bowl and toss until they are evenly coated with the honey mixture.
4. Place the carrots in a single layer on a baking sheet lined with parchment paper.
5. Roast the carrots for 20-25 minutes, stirring occasionally, until they are tender and lightly caramelized.
6. Alternatively, you can steam the carrots in a steamer basket over simmering water for 10-15 minutes or until tender.
7. Serve the carrots hot and enjoy!

Nutritional Values: Calories: 107 kcal Fat: 7g Carbohydrates: 12g Fiber: 3g Protein: 1g Sodium: 58mg

Roasted Beets with Goat Cheese

Preparation time: 15 minutes **Cooking Time:** 45 minutes **Servings:** 4
Ingredients:

- 4 medium-sized beets, peeled and cut into 1-inch cubes.
- 1 tablespoon olive oil
- Salt and black pepper, to taste
- 2 ounces crumbled goat cheese
- 1/4 cup chopped walnuts.
- 2 tablespoons chopped fresh parsley.

Instructions:

1. Preheat the oven to 400°F.

2. In a large bowl, toss the beet cubes with olive oil, salt, and black pepper until well-coated.

3. Spread the beet cubes out in a single layer on a baking sheet. Roast in the oven for 35-45 minutes, or until tender and lightly browned, stirring once halfway through.

4. In a small bowl, combine the crumbled goat cheese and chopped walnuts.

5. To serve, place the roasted beets in a bowl and top with the goat cheese and walnut mixture. Garnish with chopped fresh parsley.

Nutritional Values: Per serving | Calories: 140kcal | Fat: 10g | Carbohydrates: 10g | Fiber: 2g | Protein: 4g | Sodium: 120mg

Quinoa and Vegetable Stuffed Bell Peppers

Preparation time: 20 minutes **Cooking Time:** 45 minutes **Servings:** 7

Ingredients:
- 7 bell peppers (any color), tops removed and seeded.
- 1 tablespoon olive oil
- 1 onion, chopped.
- 2 cloves garlic, minced.
- 2 zucchinis, diced.
- 1 yellow squash, diced.
- 1 red bell pepper, diced.
- 1 cup quinoa, cooked.
- 1 teaspoon dried oregano
- 1 teaspoon dried basil
- 1/4 teaspoon salt
- 1/4 teaspoon black pepper
- 1/4 cup grated Parmesan cheese.

Instructions:
1. Preheat the oven to 375°F (190°C).
2. In a large skillet, heat the olive oil over medium heat.
3. Add the onion and garlic and sauté until soft and fragrant, about 3 minutes.
4. Add the zucchini, yellow squash, and red bell pepper to the skillet and cook until the vegetables are tender, about 8-10 minutes.
5. Add the cooked quinoa, dried oregano, dried basil, salt, and black pepper to the skillet and stir to combine.
6. Spoon the quinoa and vegetable mixture into the bell peppers, filling each pepper to the top.
7. Sprinkle the grated Parmesan cheese over the stuffed peppers.
8. Place the stuffed peppers in a baking dish and bake for 30-35 minutes, or until the peppers are tender and the cheese is melted and golden brown.
9. Serve the stuffed peppers hot.

Nutritional Values: Calories: 267 Fat: 8.3g Saturated Fat: 2.4g Sodium: 240mg Carbohydrates: 42.2g Fiber: 8.3g Sugar: 10.6g Protein: 10.1g

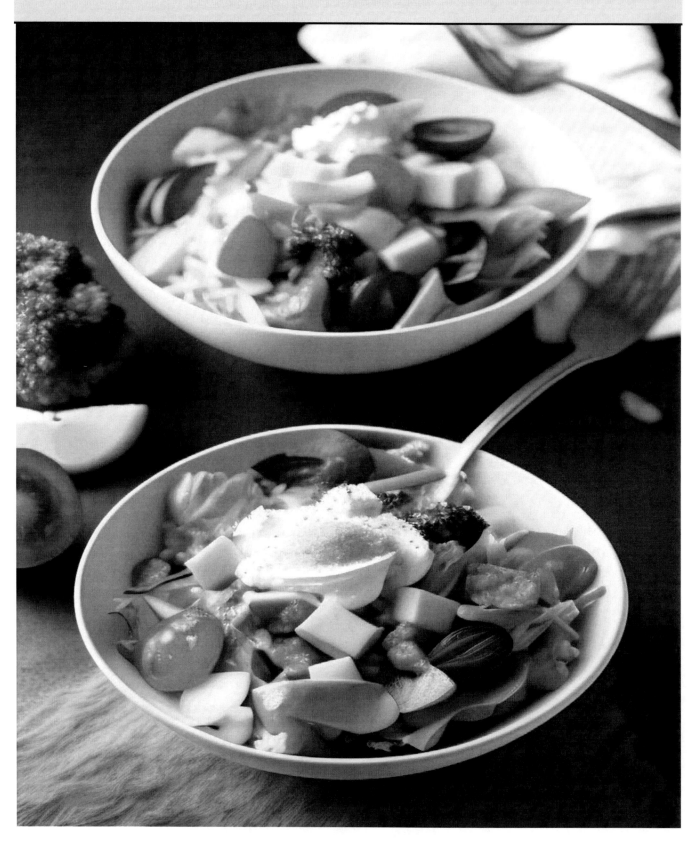

Quinoa Salad with Roasted Vegetables

Preparation time: 15 minutes **Cooking Time:** 30 minutes **Servings:** 4

Ingredients:

- 1 cup quinoa
- 2 cups mixed vegetables (such as bell peppers, zucchini, eggplant, and red onion)
- 1 tablespoon olive oil
- 1/2 teaspoon dried oregano
- 1/2 teaspoon dried thyme
- Salt and pepper to taste
- 2 tablespoons lemon juice
- 2 tablespoons olive oil
- 1/4 cup crumbled feta cheese
- Fresh parsley for garnish

Instructions:

1. Preheat the oven to 400°F (200°C).
2. Rinse the quinoa in a fine mesh strainer and place in a medium saucepan with 2 cups of water. Bring to a boil over high heat, then reduce the heat to low and cover the saucepan. Cook for 15-20 minutes, until the water is absorbed, and the quinoa is tender. Fluff with a fork and set aside.
3. Cut the mixed vegetables into bite-sized pieces and toss with 1 tablespoon of olive oil, dried oregano, dried thyme, salt, and pepper. Spread the vegetables out in a single layer on a baking sheet and roast for 20-25 minutes, until tender and lightly browned.
4. In a small bowl, whisk together the lemon juice and 2 tablespoons of olive oil.
5. In a large mixing bowl, combine the cooked quinoa, roasted vegetables, and lemon vinaigrette. Toss well to coat.
6. Divide the quinoa salad into 4 bowls and top with crumbled feta cheese and fresh parsley.

Nutritional Values: Calories: 280 kcal Fat: 14 g Carbohydrates: 32 g Fiber: 6 g Protein: 8 g Sodium: 120 mg

Lentil and Vegetable Salad

Preparation time: 15 minutes **Cooking Time:** 30 minutes **Servings:** 4

Ingredients:

- 1 cup dry lentils rinsed and drained.
- 2 cups water
- 1 red bell pepper, diced.
- 1 yellow bell pepper, diced.
- 1 small red onion, diced.
- 1/4 cup chopped fresh parsley.
- 1/4 cup chopped fresh mint.
- 1/4 cup balsamic vinegar
- 1/4 cup extra-virgin olive oil
- 2 garlic cloves, minced.
- Salt and freshly ground black pepper to taste.
- Mixed salad greens, for serving.

Instructions:

1. In a medium saucepan, combine the lentils and water. Bring to a boil, then reduce the heat and simmer until the lentils are tender, about 20 to 25 minutes. Drain and set aside.
2. In a large bowl, combine the cooked lentils, red and yellow bell peppers, red onion, parsley, and mint.
3. In a small bowl, whisk together the balsamic vinegar, olive oil, garlic, salt, and pepper.
4. Pour the dressing over the lentil and vegetable mixture and toss to combine.
5. Serve the salad over a bed of mixed salad greens.

Nutritional Values: Calories: 268kcal Fat: 14g Carbohydrates: 26g Fiber: 9g Protein: 10g Sodium: 47mg

Cobb Salad with Hard-Boiled Eggs

Preparation time: 20 minutes **Cooking Time:** 10 minutes **Servings:** 4

Ingredients:

- 8 cups mixed greens
- 2 grilled chicken breasts, sliced.

- 4 hard-boiled eggs peeled and sliced.
- 1 avocado, sliced.
- 1/2 cup cherry tomatoes, halved.
- 1/2 cup crumbled blue cheese.
- 4 slices cooked bacon, crumbled.
- 1/4 cup chopped fresh chives.
- 2 tablespoons olive oil
- 2 tablespoons red wine vinegar
- 1 teaspoon Dijon mustard
- Salt and pepper to taste

Instructions:

1. In a large bowl, combine the mixed greens, grilled chicken, hard-boiled eggs, avocado, cherry tomatoes, blue cheese, bacon, and chives.
2. In a small bowl, whisk together the olive oil, red wine vinegar, Dijon mustard, salt, and pepper.
3. Drizzle the dressing over the salad and toss to combine.
4. Serve immediately.

Nutritional Values: Calories: 430 Fat: 28g Saturated Fat: 7g Cholesterol: 245mg Sodium: 660mg Carbohydrates: 13g Fiber: 8g Sugar: 2g Protein: 33g

Caprese Salad

Preparation time: 10 minutes **Cooking Time:** N/A **Servings:** 4

Ingredients:

- 4 medium-sized ripe tomatoes, sliced.
- 8 oz fresh mozzarella cheese, sliced.
- 1/4 cup fresh basil leaves, torn.
- 2 tbsp. extra-virgin olive oil
- 1 tbsp. balsamic vinegar
- Salt and pepper to taste

Instructions:

1. Arrange the sliced tomatoes and mozzarella cheese on a large plate, alternating between them.
2. Sprinkle torn basil leaves over the top.
3. Drizzle with extra-virgin olive oil and balsamic vinegar.
4. Season with salt and pepper to taste.

5. Serve and enjoy!

Nutritional Values: Calories: 202 kcal Fat: 16.5 g Carbohydrates: 5.3 g Protein: 10 g Sodium: 236 mg Potassium: 286 mg Fiber: 1.1 g

Greek Salad with Feta Cheese

Preparation time: 15 minutes **Cooking Time:** 0 minutes **Servings:** 6

Ingredients:

- 6 cups mixed greens
- 1 cucumber, diced.
- 1 bell pepper, diced.
- 1 red onion thinly sliced.
- 1/2 cup kalamata olives, pitted.
- 4 ounces crumbled feta cheese
- 2 tablespoons extra-virgin olive oil
- 2 tablespoons red wine vinegar
- 1 teaspoon dried oregano
- Salt and black pepper, to taste

Instructions:

1. In a large bowl, combine the mixed greens, diced cucumber, diced bell pepper, thinly sliced red onion, and pitted kalamata olives.
2. In a small bowl, whisk together the extra-virgin olive oil, red wine vinegar, dried oregano, and salt and black pepper to taste.
3. Drizzle the dressing over the salad and toss to combine.
4. Sprinkle the crumbled feta cheese over the top of the salad and serve.

Nutritional Values: Calories: 223 Fat: 18g Saturated Fat: 6g Sodium: 481mg Carbohydrates: 9g Fiber: 3g Sugar: 4g Protein: 7g

Spinach and Strawberry Salad

Preparation time: 15 minutes **Cooking Time:** 0 minutes **Servings:** 4

Ingredients:

- 6 cups baby spinach leaves
- 1-pint strawberries, hulled and sliced
- 1/2 cup sliced almonds.
- 1/2 cup crumbled feta cheese
- 2 tablespoons balsamic vinegar
- 1 tablespoon honey
- 1/4 cup extra-virgin olive oil

- Salt and freshly ground black pepper to taste.

Instructions:

1. In a large bowl, combine the spinach, strawberries, almonds, and feta cheese.
2. In a small bowl, whisk together the balsamic vinegar, honey, and olive oil. Season with salt and pepper to taste.
3. Drizzle the dressing over the salad and toss to coat evenly.
4. Serve immediately.

Nutritional Values: Calories: 250 kcal Protein: 7g Fat: 21g Carbohydrates: 13g Fiber: 4g Sodium: 290mg

Kale and Quinoa Salad

Preparation time: 15 minutes **Cooking Time:** 25 minutes **Servings:** 4

Ingredients:

- 1 large, sweet potato, peeled and diced.
- 2 tablespoons olive oil
- Salt and pepper, to taste
- 1/2 cup uncooked quinoa rinsed and drained.
- 1 bunch kale, stems removed, and leaves chopped.
- 1 avocado, diced.
- 1/4 cup crumbled feta cheese
- 2 tablespoons red wine vinegar
- 1 tablespoon Dijon mustard
- 1 tablespoon honey
- 1/4 cup olive oil
- Salt and pepper, to taste

Instructions:

1. Preheat the oven to 400°F (200°C).
2. Toss the sweet potato with the olive oil, salt, and pepper. Spread the sweet potato in a single layer on a baking sheet and roast for 20-25 minutes or until tender and lightly browned.
3. While the sweet potato is roasting, cook the quinoa according to the package instructions. Once cooked, fluff with a fork and set aside.
4. In a large bowl, add the chopped kale, avocado, and feta cheese.

5. In a small bowl, whisk together the red wine vinegar, Dijon mustard, honey, olive oil, salt, and pepper.
6. Add the cooked quinoa and roasted sweet potato to the bowl with the kale mixture.
7. Pour the dressing over the salad and toss well to combine.
8. Serve the salad immediately or store in the fridge until ready to eat.

Nutritional Values: Calories: 390 kcal Protein: 9 g Fat: 26 g Carbohydrates: 34 g Fiber: 7 g Sodium: 320 mg

Black Bean and Corn Salad

Preparation time: 15 minutes **Cooking Time:** 0 minutes **Servings:** 4

Ingredients:

- **For the salad:**
- 1 can black beans, drained and rinsed.
- 1 cup frozen corn, thawed.
- 1 red bell pepper, chopped.
- 1/4 cup red onion, chopped.
- 1 jalapeno pepper seeded and chopped.
- 1/4 cup fresh cilantro, chopped.
- Salt and pepper, to taste
- 4 cups mixed greens
- **For the dressing:**
- 2 tablespoons olive oil
- 2 tablespoons fresh lime juice
- 1 tablespoon honey
- 1/4 cup fresh cilantro, chopped.
- Salt and pepper, to taste

Instructions:

1. In a large bowl, combine the black beans, corn, red bell pepper, red onion, jalapeno pepper, and cilantro. Toss to combine.
2. In a separate small bowl, whisk together the olive oil, lime juice, honey, and cilantro. Season with salt and pepper to taste.
3. Pour the dressing over the salad and toss to coat.
4. Serve the salad over a bed of mixed greens.

Nutritional Values: Calories: 216 kcal Fat: 8.5 g Saturated fat: 1.3 g Carbohydrates: 31.5 g Fiber: 7.2

g Sugar: 9.1 g Protein: 7.2 g Sodium: 128 mg

Watermelon and Feta Salad with Balsamic Glaze

Preparation time: 15 minutes **Servings:** 4
Ingredients:
- 4 cups cubed watermelon.
- 2 oz. crumbled feta cheese
- 1/4 cup chopped fresh mint leaves.
- 1/4 cup balsamic glaze
- 1 tbsp. extra-virgin olive oil
- Salt and pepper to taste

Instructions:
1. In a large bowl, combine watermelon, feta cheese, and mint leaves.
2. In a small bowl, whisk together balsamic glaze, olive oil, salt, and pepper.
3. Drizzle the dressing over the salad and toss to combine.
4. Serve immediately.

Nutritional Values: Calories: 115 Fat: 6g Carbohydrates: 14g Protein: 3g Sodium: 207mg Fiber: 1g

Beet and Goat Cheese Salad with Walnuts

Preparation time: 20 minutes **Cooking Time:** 50 minutes **Servings:** 4
Ingredients:
- 4 medium beets peeled and diced.
- 2 tablespoons olive oil, divided.
- 2 teaspoons balsamic vinegar
- 1/4 teaspoon salt
- 1/4 teaspoon black pepper
- 6 cups mixed greens
- 1/2 cup crumbled goat cheese
- 1/2 cup chopped walnuts.
- 2 tablespoons chopped fresh parsley.
- For the dressing:
- 1/4 cup olive oil
- 2 tablespoons balsamic vinegar
- 1 tablespoon honey
- 1 teaspoon Dijon mustard
- Salt and pepper to taste

Instructions:
1. Preheat the oven to 400°F (200°C).
2. In a bowl, toss the diced beets with 1 tablespoon olive oil, balsamic vinegar, salt, and pepper until coated.
3. Spread the beets in a single layer on a baking sheet and roast for 40-50 minutes, or until tender and lightly caramelized. Set aside to cool.
4. In a small bowl, whisk together the remaining 1 tablespoon of olive oil, balsamic vinegar, honey, Dijon mustard, salt, and pepper to make the dressing.
5. In a large bowl, toss the mixed greens with the dressing until coated.
6. Divide the dressed greens onto four plates.
7. Top each plate with the roasted beets, crumbled goat cheese, chopped walnuts, and chopped fresh parsley.

Nutritional Values: Calories: 314 kcal Fat: 26.1g Carbohydrates: 16.8g Fiber: 4.4g Protein: 8.4g

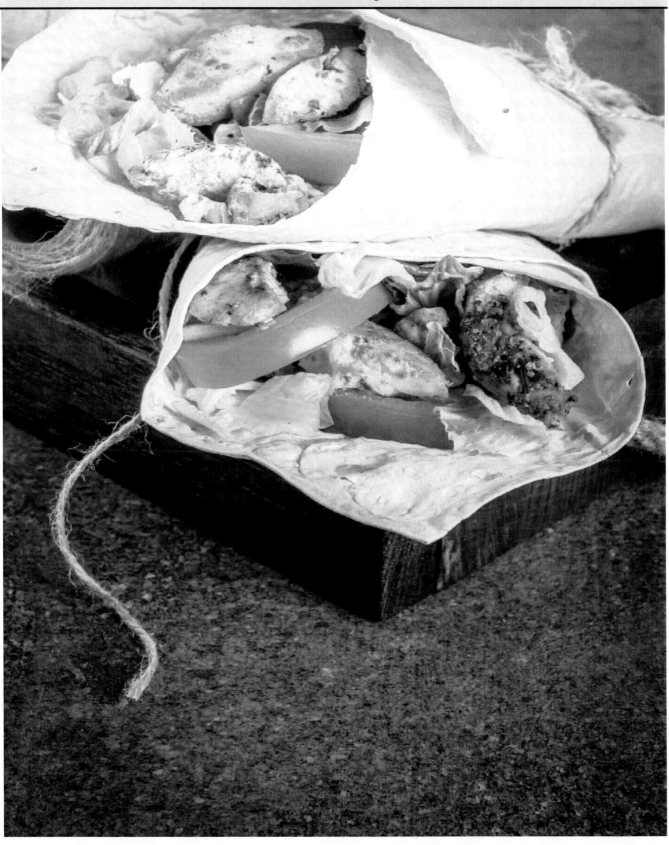

Grilled Chicken Breasts

Preparation time: 10 minutes **Cooking Time:** 20 minutes **Servings:** 4

Ingredients:

- 4 boneless, skinless chicken breasts
- 1 large red bell pepper, sliced.
- 1 large yellow onion, sliced.
- 1 large zucchini, sliced.
- 1 large yellow squash, sliced.
- 1 tbsp. olive oil
- 1 tbsp. balsamic vinegar
- 1 tbsp. dried Italian seasoning
- Salt and black pepper, to taste

Instructions:

1. Preheat the grill to medium-high heat.
2. Mix the sliced vegetables, olive oil, balsamic vinegar, Italian seasoning, salt, and black pepper in a large bowl.
3. Season the chicken breasts with salt and black pepper.
4. Place chicken breasts and vegetable mixture onto the grill. Grill chicken for 6-7 minutes per side or until fully cooked (internal temperature should reach 165°F). Grill vegetables for 8-10 minutes or until tender and lightly charred.
5. Remove chicken and vegetables from the grill and let rest for 5 minutes.
6. Serve chicken breasts with a side of mixed grilled vegetables.

Nutritional Values: Calories: 235 Total fat: 8g Saturated fat: 1g Cholesterol: 74mg Sodium: 105mg Total carbohydrate: 11g Dietary fiber: 3g Sugars: 6g Protein: 31g

Baked Turkey Meatballs with Whole-Grain Pasta

Preparation time: 20 minutes **Cooking Time:** 25 minutes **Servings:** 4

Ingredients:

- For the meatballs:
- 1 lb. lean ground turkey
- 1/2 cup whole-grain breadcrumbs
- 1 egg

- 2 tbsp. grated Parmesan cheese
- 1 tbsp. dried parsley
- 1/2 tsp garlic powder
- 1/2 tsp salt
- 1/4 tsp black pepper
- For the pasta and sauce:
- 8 oz. whole-grain spaghetti
- 2 cups low-sodium tomato sauce
- 1/2 tsp dried oregano
- 1/2 tsp dried basil
- 1/4 tsp red pepper flakes
- Salt and black pepper, to taste

Instructions:

1. Preheat oven to 400°F. Line a baking sheet with parchment paper.
2. Combine the ground turkey, breadcrumbs, egg, Parmesan cheese, parsley, garlic powder, salt, and black pepper in a large bowl. Mix until well combined.
3. Place the mixture into a 1 1/2-inch meatball on the prepared baking sheet.
4. Bake the meatballs for 20-25 minutes or until fully cooked (internal temperature should reach 165°F).
5. While the meatballs are baking, cook the whole-grain spaghetti according to the package instructions.
6. In a saucepan, heat the tomato sauce over medium heat. Add the oregano, basil, red pepper flakes, salt, and black pepper. Simmer for 5-10 minutes or until heated through.
7. Serve the meatballs over the whole-grain spaghetti, topped with tomato sauce.

Nutritional Values: Calories: 426 Total fat: 11g Saturated fat: 3g Cholesterol: 128mg Sodium: 577mg Total carbohydrate: 46g Dietary fiber: 8g Sugars: 9g Protein: 38g

Grilled Chicken with Lemon and Herbs

Preparation time: 15 minutes **Cooking Time:** 35 minutes **Servings:** 4

Ingredients:

- For the chicken:

- 4 boneless, skinless chicken breasts
- 2 tbsp. olive oil
- 1 tbsp. dried basil
- 1 tbsp. dried thyme
- 1 tbsp. dried oregano
- 1 lemon, juiced.
- Salt and black pepper, to taste

For the sweet potatoes and green beans:
- 2 large, sweet potatoes, peeled and diced.
- 1 lb. fresh green beans, trimmed.
- 2 tbsp. olive oil
- 1 tsp garlic powder
- 1 tsp paprika
- Salt and black pepper, to taste

Instructions:
1. Preheat the grill to medium-high heat.
2. Mix the olive oil, dried herbs, lemon juice, salt, and black pepper in a small bowl. Brush the chicken breasts with the mixture.
3. Place the chicken breasts onto the grill. Grill for 6-7 minutes per side or until fully cooked (internal temperature should reach 165°F).
4. While the chicken is grilling, preheat the oven to 425°F. Line a baking sheet with parchment paper.
5. Toss the diced sweet potatoes, green beans, olive oil, garlic powder, paprika, salt, and black pepper in a large bowl. Spread the mixture onto the prepared baking sheet.
6. Roast the sweet potatoes and green beans for 20-25 minutes or until tender and lightly browned.
7. Serve the grilled chicken breasts with roasted sweet potatoes and green beans.

Nutritional Values: Calories: 406 Total fat: 17g Saturated fat: 3g Cholesterol: 96mg Sodium: 143mg Total carbohydrate: 28g Dietary fiber: 7g Sugars: 8g Protein: 38g

Baked Chicken Thighs

Preparation time: 15 minutes **Cooking Time:** 45 minutes **Servings:** 4
Ingredients:
- For the chicken:

- 4 bone-in, skin-on chicken thighs
- 1 tbsp. olive oil
- 1 tsp garlic powder
- 1 tsp dried thyme
- Salt and black pepper, to taste

For the Brussels sprouts and carrots:
- 1 lb. Brussels sprouts trimmed and halved.
- 4 large carrots peeled and sliced.
- 1 tbsp. olive oil
- 1 tsp garlic powder
- 1 tsp dried thyme
- Salt and black pepper, to taste

Instructions:
1. Preheat oven to 375°F. Line a baking sheet with parchment paper.
2. Mix the olive oil, garlic powder, dried thyme, salt, and black pepper in a small bowl. Brush the chicken thighs with the mixture.
3. Place the chicken thighs onto the prepared baking sheet.
4. Toss the halved Brussels sprouts, sliced carrots, olive oil, garlic powder, dried thyme, salt, and black pepper in a large bowl. Spread the mixture onto the prepared baking sheet around the chicken thighs.
5. Bake for 40-45 minutes until the chicken is fully cooked (internal temperature should reach 165°F) and the vegetables are tender and lightly browned.
6. Serve the baked chicken thighs with roasted Brussels sprouts and carrots.

Nutritional Values: Calories: 364 Total fat: 19g Saturated fat: 4g Cholesterol: 113mg Sodium: 184mg Total carbohydrate: 20g Dietary fiber: 7g Sugars: 7g Protein: 29g

Turkey Meatloaf

Preparation time: 15 minutes **Cooking Time:** 1-hour **Servings:** 6
Ingredients:
For the meatloaf:
- 2 lbs. ground turkey
- 1/2 cup whole-grain breadcrumbs
- 1/2 cup unsweetened almond milk

- 2 eggs
- 1 small onion finely chopped.
- 1 tbsp. dried rosemary
- 1 tsp garlic powder
- 1 tsp salt
- 1/2 tsp black pepper
- 1/2 cup low-sodium tomato sauce

For the cauliflower and carrots:
- 1 head cauliflower, cut into florets.
- 4 large carrots peeled and sliced.
- 2 tbsp. olive oil
- 1 tbsp. dried rosemary
- Salt and black pepper, to taste

Instructions:

1. Preheat oven to 375°F. Line a baking sheet with parchment paper.
2. Combine the ground turkey, breadcrumbs, almond milk, eggs, onion, dried rosemary, garlic powder, salt, and black pepper in a large bowl. Mix until well combined.
3. Transfer the mixture to a loaf pan. Spread the tomato sauce over the top of the meatloaf.
4. Bake the meatloaf for 50-60 minutes or until fully cooked (internal temperature should reach 165°F).
5. While the meatloaf is baking, preheat the oven to 425°F. Line a baking sheet with parchment paper.
6. Toss the cauliflower florets, sliced carrots, olive oil, dried rosemary, salt, and black pepper in a large bowl. Spread the mixture onto the prepared baking sheet.
7. Roast the cauliflower and carrots for 20-25 minutes or until tender and lightly browned.
8. Serve the turkey meatloaf with a side of roasted cauliflower and carrots.

Nutritional Values: Calories: 357 Total fat: 15g Saturated fat: 4g Cholesterol: 181mg Sodium: 662mg Total carbohydrate: 21g Dietary fiber: 6g Sugars: 6g Protein: 36g

Chicken and Vegetable Fajita Bowl with Quinoa

Preparation time: 15 minutes **Cooking Time:** 25 minutes **Servings:** 4

Ingredients:

For the chicken and vegetables:
- 1 lb. boneless, skinless chicken breast sliced into thin strips.
- 2 bell peppers, seeded and cut into thin strips.
- 1 large onion, cut into thin strips.
- 2 tbsp. olive oil
- 1 tbsp. chili powder
- 1 tsp ground cumin
- 1/2 tsp garlic powder
- Salt and black pepper, to taste

For the quinoa:
- 1 cup quinoa, rinsed.
- 2 cups water
- 1/2 tsp salt
- For the mixed greens:
- 4 cups mixed greens
- 2 tbsp. balsamic vinegar
- 1 tbsp. olive oil

Instructions:

1. Preheat oven to 400°F. Line a baking sheet with parchment paper.
2. In a large bowl, toss together the chicken strips, sliced bell peppers, sliced onion, olive oil, chili powder, ground cumin, garlic powder, salt, and black pepper.
3. Spread the mixture onto the prepared baking sheet.
4. Bake for 20-25 minutes until the chicken is fully cooked and the vegetables are tender and lightly browned.
5. While the chicken and vegetables are baking, prepare the quinoa. Bring the rinsed quinoa, water, and salt to a boil in a medium saucepan. Reduce heat to low, cover, and simmer for 15-20 minutes or until the water is fully absorbed and the quinoa is tender.
6. Toss the mixed greens, balsamic vinegar, and olive oil in a large bowl.

7. Divide the quinoa among 4 bowls. Top each bowl with the chicken and vegetable mixture and mixed greens.

Nutritional Values: Calories: 375 Total fat: 14g Saturated fat: 2g Cholesterol: 74mg Sodium: 398mg Total carbohydrate: 36g Dietary fiber: 7g Sugars: 7g Protein: 29g

Grilled Chicken Caesar Salad

Preparation time: 20 minutes **Cooking Time:** 20 minutes **Servings:** 4

Ingredients:

For the chicken:
- 4 boneless, skinless chicken breasts
- 1 tbsp. olive oil
- 1 tsp garlic powder
- Salt and black pepper, to taste
- For the salad:
- 8 cups chopped romaine lettuce.
- 1/2 cup freshly grated Parmesan cheese.
- 1/2 cup whole-grain croutons.
- 1/4 cup chopped fresh parsley.

For the dressing:
- 1/2 cup plain Greek yogurt.
- 2 tbsp. freshly squeezed lemon juice.
- 2 tbsp. Dijon mustard
- 2 tbsp. grated Parmesan cheese
- 1 tbsp. Worcestershire sauce
- 1 tsp garlic powder
- Salt and black pepper, to taste
- For the bread:
- 4 slices whole-grain bread
- 1 tbsp. olive oil
- 1 tsp garlic powder

Instructions:

1. Preheat the grill to medium-high heat.
2. Brush the chicken breasts with olive oil and season with garlic powder, salt, and black pepper.
3. Grill the chicken for 6-7 minutes per side or until fully cooked (internal temperature should reach 165°F). Set aside.
4. Combine the chopped romaine lettuce, freshly grated Parmesan cheese, whole-grain croutons, and chopped fresh parsley in a large bowl.
5. Whisk together the plain Greek yogurt, freshly squeezed lemon juice, Dijon mustard, grated Parmesan cheese, Worcestershire sauce, garlic powder, salt, and black pepper in a small bowl.
6. Heat a non-stick skillet over medium heat. Brush the slices of whole-grain bread with olive oil and sprinkle with garlic powder. Toast the bread in the skillet until lightly browned on both sides.
7. Divide the salad among 4 plates. Top each dish with grilled chicken breast and drizzle with the homemade dressing. Serve with a slice of whole-grain bread on the side.

Nutritional Values: Calories: 401 Total fat: 16g Saturated fat: 4g Cholesterol: 99mg Sodium: 697mg Total carbohydrate: 29g Dietary fiber: 5g Sugars: 5g Protein: 36g

Chicken and Vegetable Lettuce Wraps

Preparation time: 20 minutes **Cooking Time:** 10 minutes **Servings:** 4

Ingredients:

For the chicken and vegetables:
- 1 lb. ground chicken
- 1 tbsp. olive oil
- 1 red bell pepper seeded and diced.
- 1 cup chopped mushrooms.
- 1 cup shredded carrots
- 2 green onions, chopped.
- 2 cloves garlic, minced.
- Salt and black pepper, to taste
- 8 large lettuce leaves

For the peanut sauce:
- 1/4 cup natural peanut butter
- 2 tbsp. low-sodium soy sauce
- 2 tbsp. rice vinegar
- 1 tbsp. honey
- 1 tbsp. sesame oil
- 1 tbsp. water
- 1/2 tsp garlic powder

- Pinch of red pepper flakes

Instructions:

1. Heat olive oil in a large skillet over medium-high heat. Add the ground chicken, red bell pepper, mushrooms, shredded carrots, green onions, and minced garlic. Cook for 7-10 minutes or until the chicken is fully cooked and the vegetables are tender.
2. Whisk together the peanut butter, low-sodium soy sauce, rice vinegar, honey, sesame oil, water, garlic powder, and red pepper flakes in a small bowl.
3. To assemble the lettuce wraps, spoon the chicken and vegetable mixture onto each lettuce leaf. Drizzle with the peanut sauce and serve.

Nutritional Values: Calories: 302 Total fat: 19g Saturated fat: 4g Cholesterol: 98mg Sodium: 478mg Total carbohydrate: 12g Dietary fiber: 3g Sugars: 6g Protein: 25g

Grilled Chicken and Vegetable Wrap

Preparation time: 20 minutes **Cooking Time:** 15 minutes **Servings:** 4
Ingredients:

For the chicken and vegetables:

- 1 lb. boneless, skinless chicken breasts
- 1 tbsp. olive oil
- 1 red bell pepper seeded and sliced.
- 1 yellow squash, sliced.
- 1 zucchini, sliced.
- 1 red onion, sliced.
- Salt and black pepper, to taste

For the wrap:

- 4 whole-wheat tortillas
- 1/2 cup hummus
- 1/4 cup crumbled feta cheese
- 1/4 cup chopped fresh parsley.
- Juice of 1/2 lemon

Instructions:

1. Preheat the grill to medium-high heat.
2. Brush the chicken breasts with olive oil and season with salt and black pepper.

3. Grill the chicken for 6-7 minutes per side or until fully cooked (internal temperature should reach 165°F). Set aside.
4. Toss the sliced red bell pepper, yellow squash, zucchini, and red onion with olive oil, salt, and black pepper in a large bowl. Grill for 5-7 minutes or until tender and slightly charred. Set aside.
5. To assemble the wrap, spread 2 tablespoons of hummus onto each tortilla. Top with sliced grilled chicken, grilled vegetables, crumbled feta cheese, chopped fresh parsley, and a squeeze of fresh lemon juice.
6. Roll up the tortilla and cut it in half diagonally. Serve immediately.

Nutritional Values: Calories: 375 Total fat: 15g Saturated fat: 4g Cholesterol: 74mg Sodium: 604mg Total carbohydrate: 31g Dietary fiber: 7g Sugars: 5g Protein: 30g

Spicy Chicken and Vegetable Stir-Fry

Preparation time: 20 minutes **Cooking Time:** 20 minutes **Servings:** 4
Ingredients:

For the stir-fry:

- 1 lb. boneless, skinless chicken breasts cut into small pieces.
- 2 tbsp. low-sodium soy sauce
- 2 tbsp. rice vinegar
- 1 tbsp. cornstarch
- 1 tbsp. sesame oil
- 2 cloves garlic, minced.
- 1 tbsp. grated fresh ginger.
- 1 red bell pepper seeded and sliced.
- 1 yellow bell pepper seeded and sliced.
- 1 cup sliced mushrooms.
- 1 cup sliced zucchini.
- 2 green onions, chopped.
- Salt and black pepper, to taste

For the brown rice:

- 1 cup brown rice
- 2 cups water
- Pinch of salt

Instructions:

1. Whisk together the low-sodium soy sauce, rice vinegar, cornstarch, and sesame oil in a small bowl. Set aside.
2. Cook the brown rice according to package instructions with a pinch of salt.
3. Heat a large skillet or wok over high heat. Add the minced garlic and grated ginger and cook for 30 seconds or until fragrant.
4. Add the chicken and cook for 5-7 minutes or until fully cooked.
5. Add the sliced bell peppers, mushrooms, and zucchini to the skillet and cook for 3-4 minutes or until tender.
6. Pour the soy sauce mixture over the chicken and vegetables and stir to coat evenly. Cook for 1-2 minutes or until the sauce thickens.
7. Serve the stir-fry over brown rice and sprinkle with chopped green onions.

Nutritional Values: Calories: 344 Total fat: 7g Saturated fat: 1g Cholesterol: 73mg Sodium: 455mg Total carbohydrate: 39g Dietary fiber: 5g Sugars: 5g Protein: 32g

Seafood

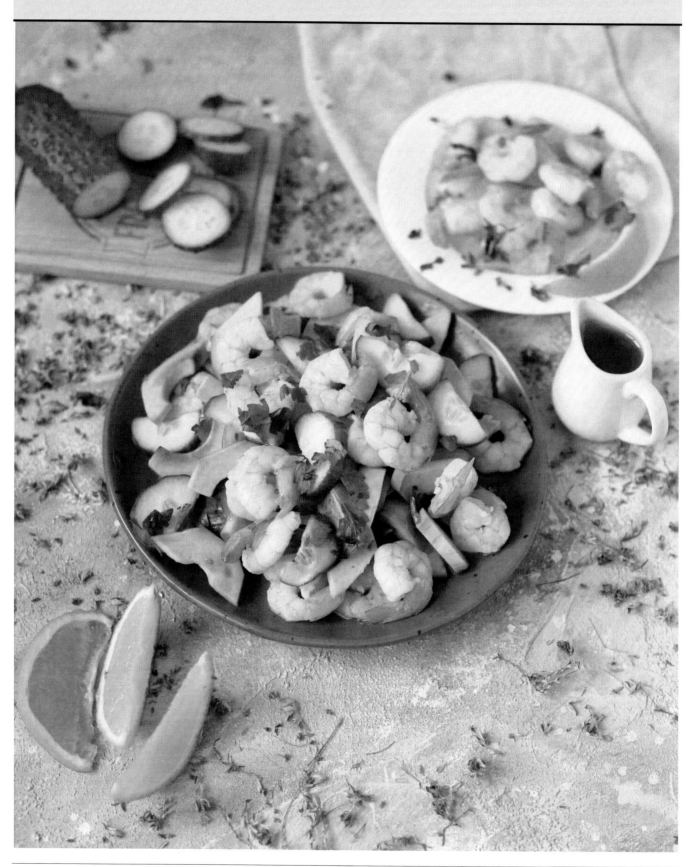

Spicy Shrimp and Vegetable Stir-Fry

Preparation time: 15 minutes **Cooking Time:** 15 minutes **Servings:** 4

Ingredients:

- For the stir-fry:
- 1 lb. large shrimp peeled and deveined.
- 2 tbsp. low-sodium soy sauce
- 1 tbsp. rice vinegar
- 1 tbsp. cornstarch
- 1 tbsp. vegetable oil
- 2 cloves garlic, minced.
- 1 tbsp. grated fresh ginger.
- 1 red bell pepper seeded and sliced.
- 1 yellow bell pepper seeded and sliced.
- 1 cup sliced mushrooms.
- 1 cup sliced zucchini.
- 2 green onions, chopped.
- Salt and black pepper, to taste
- Crushed red pepper flakes to taste.
- For the brown rice:
- 1 cup brown rice
- 2 cups water
- Pinch of salt

Instructions:

1. Whisk together the low-sodium soy sauce, rice vinegar, cornstarch, and vegetable oil in a small bowl. Set aside.
2. Cook the brown rice according to package instructions with a pinch of salt.
3. Heat a large skillet or wok over high heat. Add the minced garlic and grated ginger and cook for 30 seconds or until fragrant.
4. Add the shrimp and cook for 2-3 minutes or until fully cooked. Remove from the skillet and set aside.
5. Add the sliced bell peppers, mushrooms, and zucchini to the skillet and cook for 3-4 minutes or until tender.
6. Return the shrimp to the skillet and pour the soy sauce mixture over the shrimp and vegetables. Stir to coat evenly. Cook for 1-2 minutes or until the sauce thickens.
7. Sprinkle with chopped green onions, salt, black pepper, and crushed red pepper flakes to taste.
8. Serve the stir-fry over brown rice.

Nutritional Values: Calories: 304 Total fat: 5g Saturated fat: 1g Cholesterol: 172mg Sodium: 645mg Total carbohydrate: 37g Dietary fiber: 4g Sugars: 4g Protein: 29g

Blackened Catfish with Collard Greens

Preparation time: 15 minutes **Cooking Time:** 35 minutes **Servings:** 4

Ingredients:

- For the catfish:
- 4 catfish fillets (4-6 ounces each)
- 1 tbsp. paprika
- 1 tsp garlic powder
- 1 tsp onion powder
- 1 tsp dried thyme
- 1 tsp dried oregano
- 1/2 tsp cayenne pepper
- 1/2 tsp black pepper
- 1/4 tsp salt
- 1 tbsp olive oil
- For the collard greens:
- 2 bunches of collard greens washed and chopped.
- 1 tbsp. olive oil
- 1/2 onion, diced.
- 2 cloves garlic, minced.
- 1/4 tsp salt
- 1/4 tsp black pepper
- 1/4 tsp red pepper flakes
- 1/2 cup low-sodium chicken broth
- For the sweet potatoes:
- 2 large, sweet potatoes, peeled and diced.
- 1 tbsp. olive oil
- 1/4 tsp salt
- 1/4 tsp black pepper

Instructions:

1. Preheat the oven to 400°F.

2. Mix the paprika, garlic powder, onion powder, dried thyme, dried oregano, cayenne pepper, black pepper, and salt in a small bowl.

3. Rub the spice mixture onto both sides of the catfish fillets.

4. Heat 1 tbsp olive oil in a large skillet over medium-high heat. Add the catfish fillets and cook for 4-5 minutes on each side until blackened and fully cooked. Remove from the skillet and set aside.

5. Heat another tablespoon of olive oil over medium-high heat in the same skillet. Add the diced onion and minced garlic and cook until fragrant, about 1-2 minutes.

6. Add the chopped collard greens, salt, black pepper, red pepper flakes, and low-sodium chicken broth. Cover and cook for 10-12 minutes or until the collard greens are tender.

7. Toss the diced sweet potatoes with 1 tbsp. olive oil, salt, and black pepper in a separate baking dish. Roast in the oven for 20-25 minutes or until tender and golden brown.

8. Serve the blackened catfish with collard greens and roasted sweet potatoes on the side.

Nutritional Values: Calories: 353 Total fat: 11g Saturated fat: 2g Cholesterol: 68mg Sodium: 434mg Total carbohydrate: 36g Dietary fiber: 8g Sugars: 9g Protein: 30g

Grilled Tuna Steak with Steamed Broccoli

Preparation time: 10 minutes **Cooking Time:** 15 minutes **Servings:** 2
Ingredients:
- 2 tuna steaks (6 ounces each)
- 1 tbsp. olive oil
- 1/2 tsp salt
- 1/4 tsp black pepper
- 1/4 tsp garlic powder
- 1/4 tsp onion powder
- 1/4 tsp dried oregano
- 1/4 tsp dried thyme

- 1 cup brown rice, cooked according to package instructions.
- 2 cups broccoli florets
- 1 tbsp. lemon juice

Instructions:
1. Preheat the grill to high heat.
2. Mix the olive oil, salt, black pepper, garlic powder, onion powder, dried oregano, and dried thyme in a small bowl.
3. Brush both sides of the tuna steaks with the olive oil mixture.
4. Grill the tuna steaks on each side for 2-3 minutes or until cooked to your desired doneness. Remove from the grill and set aside.
5. In a separate pot, steam the broccoli florets for 5-7 minutes or until tender.
6. Serve the grilled tuna steak with steamed broccoli and brown rice. Squeeze some fresh lemon juice over the broccoli before serving.

Nutritional Values: Calories: 406 Total fat: 11g Saturated fat: 2g Cholesterol: 68mg Sodium: 652mg Total carbohydrate: 45g Dietary fiber: 6g Sugars: 2g Protein: 36g

Baked Cod with Roasted Mixed Vegetables

Preparation time: 10 minutes **Cooking Time:** 25 minutes **Servings:** 4
Ingredients:
- 4 cod fillets (4-6 ounces each)
- 1 tbsp. olive oil
- 1/2 tsp salt
- 1/4 tsp black pepper
- 1/4 tsp garlic powder
- 1/4 tsp onion powder
- 1/4 tsp dried oregano
- 1/4 tsp dried thyme
- 2 cups mixed vegetables (such as bell peppers, zucchini, and onion), chopped.
- 1 cup cooked quinoa

Instructions:
1. Preheat the oven to 400°F.

2. Line a baking sheet with parchment paper or aluminum foil.

3. Place the cod fillets on the prepared baking sheet.

4. Mix the olive oil, salt, black pepper, garlic powder, onion powder, dried oregano, and dried thyme in a small bowl.

5. Brush both sides of the cod fillets with the olive oil mixture.

6. Scatter the mixed vegetables around the cod fillets on the baking sheet.

7. Bake in the preheated oven for 20-25 minutes, or until the cod is cooked through and the vegetables are tender.

8. Serve the baked cod with roasted mixed vegetables and cooked quinoa.

Nutritional Values: Calories: 221 Total fat: 7g Saturated fat: 1g Cholesterol: 50mg Sodium: 400mg Total carbohydrate: 14g Dietary fiber: 3g Sugars: 2g Protein: 25g

Shrimp and Vegetable Curry with Brown Rice

Preparation time: 15 minutes **Cooking Time:** 20 minutes **Servings:** 4

Ingredients:

- 1 tbsp olive oil
- 1 onion, chopped.
- 2 cloves garlic, minced.
- 1 tbsp ginger, minced.
- 1 red bell pepper, chopped.
- 1 zucchini, chopped.
- 1 cup cherry tomatoes, halved.
- 1 tbsp curry powder
- 1/2 tsp salt
- 1/4 tsp black pepper
- 1/4 tsp cumin
- 1 lb. raw shrimp peeled and deveined.
- 2 cups cooked brown rice.
- 4 cups fresh spinach

Instructions:

1. Heat the olive oil in a large skillet over medium heat.

2. Add the onion, garlic, and ginger to the skillet and cook until the onion is translucent about 3-4 minutes.

3. Add the red bell pepper and zucchini to the skillet and cook for 3-4 minutes, until the vegetables are tender.

4. Add the cherry tomatoes, curry powder, salt, black pepper, and cumin to the skillet and stir to combine.

5. Add the raw shrimp to the skillet until the shrimp are pink and cooked through, about 5-7 minutes.

6. While the shrimp and vegetables are cooking, steam the spinach until wilted.

7. Serve the shrimp and vegetable curry over a bed of cooked brown rice with steamed spinach.

Nutritional Values: Calories: 311 Total fat: 7g Saturated fat: 1g Cholesterol: 172mg Sodium: 571mg Total carbohydrate: 32g Dietary fiber: 5g Sugars: 6g Protein: 29g

Lemon and Herb Baked Salmon

Preparation time: 10 minutes **Cooking Time:** 20 minutes **Servings:** 4

Ingredients:

- 4 salmon fillets
- 2 tbsp. olive oil
- 1 tbsp. fresh lemon juice
- 1 tbsp. fresh parsley, chopped.
- 1 tbsp. fresh dill, chopped.
- Salt and pepper, to taste
- 1 lb. green beans, trimmed.
- 1 cup cooked quinoa

Instructions:

1. Preheat the oven to 375°F.

2. Whisk together the olive oil, lemon juice, parsley, dill, salt, and pepper in a small bowl.

3. Place the salmon fillets in a baking dish and spoon the lemon and herb mixture over the top of the fillets.

4. Bake the salmon in the oven for 15-20 minutes or until the salmon is cooked through and flakes easily with a fork.

5. While the salmon is baking, spread the green beans on a baking sheet and drizzle with olive oil, salt, and pepper.
6. Roast the green beans in the oven for 10-15 minutes or until tender and slightly browned.
7. Serve the baked salmon with a side of roasted green beans and quinoa.

Nutritional Values: Calories: 402 Total fat: 20g Saturated fat: 3g Cholesterol: 85mg Sodium: 126mg Total carbohydrate: 18g Dietary fiber: 5g Sugars: 4g Protein: 38g

Grilled Seafood and Vegetable Kabobs

Preparation time: 20 minutes **Cooking Time:** 10-15 minutes **Servings:** 4
Ingredients:

- 1 lb. shrimp peeled and deveined.
- 1 lb. scallops
- 2 zucchinis, sliced into rounds.
- 1 red onion, cut into chunks.
- 1 red bell pepper, cut into chunks.
- 1 yellow bell pepper, cut into chunks.
- 1/4 cup olive oil
- 2 tbsp fresh lemon juice
- 2 cloves garlic, minced.
- Salt and pepper, to taste
- 2 cups cooked brown rice.
- 2 tbsp fresh parsley, chopped.

Instructions:

1. Soak wooden skewers in water for at least 30 minutes.
2. Preheat the grill to medium-high heat.
3. Thread the shrimp, scallops, zucchini, onion, and bell peppers onto the skewers.
4. Whisk together the olive oil, lemon juice, garlic, salt, and pepper in a small bowl.
5. Brush the kabobs with the olive oil mixture.
6. Grill the kabobs for 10-15 minutes, turning occasionally, or until the seafood is cooked and the vegetables are tender.
7. While the kabobs are grilling, prepare the brown rice pilaf by stirring the chopped parsley into the cooked brown rice.

8. Serve the grilled seafood and vegetable kabobs with a side of brown rice pilaf.

Nutritional Values: Calories: 458 Total fat: 18g Saturated fat: 3g Cholesterol: 216mg Sodium: 262mg Total carbohydrate: 41g Dietary fiber: 5g Sugars: 6g Protein: 36g

Baked Lemon and Herb Tilapia

Preparation time: 15 minutes **Cooking Time:** 25-30 minutes **Servings:** 4
Ingredients:

- 4 tilapia fillets
- 1 lemon, sliced.
- 2 tbsp. olive oil
- 2 tbsp. fresh parsley, chopped.
- 1 tbsp. fresh thyme, chopped.
- 1 tbsp. fresh rosemary, chopped.
- Salt and pepper, to taste
- 4 medium-sized carrots, peeled and cut into chunks.
- 4 medium-sized parsnips, peeled and cut into chunks.
- 1 medium-sized sweet potato, peeled and cut into chunks.
- 2 tbsp. olive oil

Instructions:

1. Preheat oven to 375°F (190°C).
2. Line a baking sheet with parchment paper.
3. Place the tilapia fillets on the baking sheet.
4. Drizzle the olive oil over the tilapia fillets.
5. Sprinkle the chopped herbs over the tilapia fillets.
6. Place a lemon slice on top of each tilapia fillet.
7. Season with salt and pepper.
8. Toss the carrot, parsnip, and sweet potato chunks in a separate bowl with olive oil, salt, and pepper.
9. Arrange the vegetable chunks around the tilapia fillets on the baking sheet.
10. Bake for 25-30 minutes or until the tilapia is cooked through and the vegetables are tender.
11. Serve the baked lemon and herb tilapia with roasted root vegetables.

Nutritional Values: Calories: 291 Total fat: 13g Saturated fat: 2g Cholesterol: 57mg Sodium: 98mg Total carbohydrate: 23g Dietary fiber: 6g Sugars: 8g Protein: 23g

Seared Sea Scallops

Preparation time: 10 minutes **Cooking Time:** 10 minutes **Servings:** 4

Ingredients:

- 1 lb. sea scallops
- 1 tbsp. olive oil
- Salt and pepper, to taste
- 4 cups mixed greens
- 2 cups cooked brown rice.
- 2 tbsp. balsamic vinegar
- 1 tbsp. honey
- 1 tsp Dijon mustard
- 1 garlic clove, minced.

Instructions:

1. Pat the sea scallops dry with a paper towel and season with salt and pepper.
2. Heat the olive oil in a large skillet over medium-high heat.
3. Once the oil is hot, add the sea scallops to the skillet.
4. Cook for 2-3 minutes on each side until golden brown and cooked through.
5. Whisk together the balsamic vinegar, honey, Dijon mustard, and minced garlic in a small bowl to make the dressing.
6. In a large bowl, toss the mixed greens with the dressing.
7. Divide the cooked brown rice among four plates.
8. Top each plate with the seared sea scallops and a portion of the mixed greens salad.

Nutritional Values: Calories: 274 Total fat: 5g Saturated fat: 1g Cholesterol: 37mg Sodium: 465mg Total carbohydrate: 34g Dietary fiber: 3g Sugars: 8g Protein: 22g

Shrimp and Vegetable Stir-Fry

Preparation time: 15 minutes **Cooking Time:** 10 minutes **Servings:** 4

Ingredients:

- 8 oz. soba noodles
- 1 lb. raw shrimp peeled and deveined.
- 1 tbsp. olive oil
- 1 red bell pepper, sliced.
- 1 cup sliced mushrooms.
- 1 cup chopped broccoli.
- 2 garlic cloves, minced.
- Salt and pepper, to taste
- 1/4 cup low-sodium soy sauce
- 2 tbsp. natural peanut butter
- 1 tbsp. honey
- 1 tbsp. rice vinegar
- 1 tsp sesame oil
- 1/4 tsp red pepper flakes
- Chopped green onions and cilantro for garnish.

Instructions:

1. Cook the soba noodles according to package instructions.
2. Drain the noodles and set them aside.
3. Heat the olive oil over medium-high heat in a large skillet or wok.
4. Add the red bell pepper, mushrooms, and broccoli to the skillet and stir-fry for 3-4 minutes until tender-crisp.
5. Add the minced garlic and shrimp to the skillet and stir-fry for 2-3 minutes until the shrimp is pink and cooked.
6. Whisk together the soy sauce, peanut butter, honey, rice vinegar, sesame oil, and red pepper flakes in a small bowl to make the peanut sauce.
7. Pour the peanut sauce over the shrimp and vegetable stir-fry and toss to coat.
8. Serve the stir-fry over the cooked soba noodles and garnish with chopped green onions and cilantro.

Nutritional Values: Calories: 385 Total fat: 8g Saturated fat: 1g Cholesterol: 172mg Sodium: 1003mg Total carbohydrate: 49g Dietary fiber: 5g

Sugars: 9g Protein: 30g

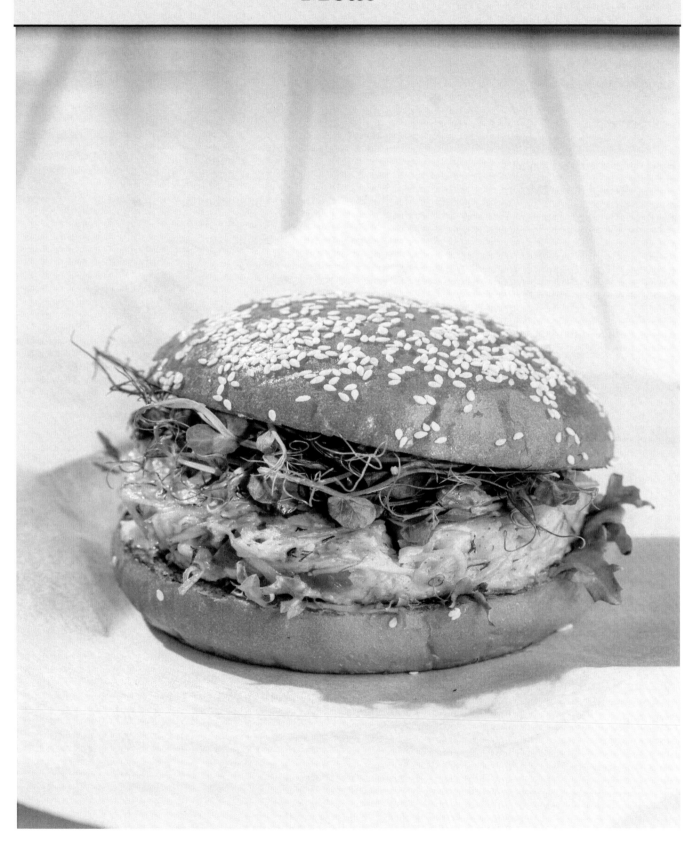

Grilled Flank Steak with Roasted Vegetables

Preparation time: 15 minutes **Cooking Time:** 25 minutes **Servings:** 4

Ingredients:

- 1-pound flank steak
- 2 cups mixed vegetables (such as bell peppers, zucchini, and onion), chopped.
- 1 tablespoon olive oil
- Salt and pepper
- 1 cup quinoa
- 2 cups water or low-sodium chicken broth
- 1 teaspoon garlic powder
- 1 teaspoon onion powder
- 1 teaspoon dried thyme

Instructions:

1. Preheat the grill to medium-high heat.
2. Season flank steak with salt and pepper.
3. Grill steak for 5-6 minutes per side for medium-rare or until the desired doneness is reached.
4. While the steak is cooking, preheat the oven to 400°F.
5. Toss mixed vegetables with olive oil and season with salt and pepper. Spread in a single layer on a baking sheet and roast in the oven for 20 minutes or until tender.
6. Combine quinoa, water or broth, garlic powder, onion powder, and thyme in a medium pot. Bring to a boil, then reduce heat and simmer for 15-20 minutes, or until liquid is absorbed and quinoa is cooked.
7. Serve sliced steak with roasted vegetables and quinoa.

Nutritional Values: Calories: 352 Fat: 10g Carbohydrates: 35g Protein: 31g Fiber: 5g Sodium: 109mg

Lemon Garlic Pork Chops

Preparation time: 10 minutes **Cooking Time:** 20 minutes **Servings:** 4

Ingredients:

- 4 boneless pork chops
- 2 tablespoons olive oil
- 2 garlic cloves, minced.
- 2 tablespoons lemon juice
- 1 tablespoon honey
- 1 teaspoon dried thyme
- 1/2 teaspoon salt
- 1/4 teaspoon black pepper
- 1 bunch of asparagus, trimmed.

Instructions:

1. Preheat the oven to 375°F (190°C).
2. Whisk together the olive oil, minced garlic, lemon juice, honey, dried thyme, salt, and black pepper in a small bowl.
3. Place the pork chops in a baking dish and brush them generously with the lemon garlic mixture.
4. Bake for 15-20 minutes or until the internal temperature of the pork chops reaches 145°F (63°C).
5. While the pork chops are baking, arrange the asparagus on a baking sheet and drizzle with any remaining lemon garlic mixture.
6. Bake the asparagus in the oven for 10-12 minutes or until tender and slightly browned.
7. Serve the pork chops with the roasted asparagus on the side.

Nutritional Values: Calories: 266 Fat: 14g Carbohydrates: 9g Protein: 26g Sodium: 388mg

Grilled Sirloin Steak

Preparation time: 10 minutes **Cooking Time:** 15 minutes **Servings:** 4

Ingredients:

- 1 lb. sirloin steak
- Salt and pepper, to taste
- 1 tbsp. olive oil
- 5 cups mixed greens
- 1 large cucumber, sliced.
- 1 cup cherry tomatoes, halved.
- 1/4 cup chopped red onion.
- 1/4 cup chopped fresh parsley.
- 2 tbsp. lemon juice
- 1 tbsp. Dijon mustard
- 1 clove garlic, minced.
- 1/4 cup olive oil

Instructions:

1. Preheat the grill to medium-high heat.
2. Season the steak with salt and pepper, then rub with 1 tablespoon olive oil.
3. Grill the steak for 6-7 minutes per side or until the desired doneness is reached. Let the steak rest for 5 minutes before slicing.
4. Combine the mixed greens, cucumber, cherry tomatoes, red onion, and parsley in a large bowl.
5. Whisk together the lemon juice, Dijon mustard, minced garlic, and 1/4 cup of olive oil in a small bowl. Season with salt and pepper to taste.
6. Drizzle the lemon dressing over the salad and toss to combine.
7. Serve the sliced steak over the salad.

Nutritional Values: Calories: 337kcal Fat: 24g Protein: 25g Carbohydrates: 7g Fiber: 2g Sugar: 3g Sodium: 154mg

Beef Stir-Fry with Brown Rice

Preparation time: 15 minutes **Cooking Time:** 20 minutes **Servings:** 4

Ingredients:

- 1-pound lean beef sirloin, sliced thinly
- 2 tablespoons low-sodium soy sauce
- 2 tablespoons rice vinegar
- 1 tablespoon honey
- 1 tablespoon cornstarch
- 2 tablespoons canola oil
- 2 garlic cloves, minced.
- 1 tablespoon grated fresh ginger.
- 2 cups mixed vegetables (such as sliced bell peppers, broccoli florets, and sliced carrots)
- 4 cups cooked brown rice.

Instructions:

1. Whisk together soy sauce, rice vinegar, honey, and cornstarch in a small bowl until well combined.
2. Heat a large wok or skillet over high heat. Add canola oil and swirl to coat.
3. Add garlic and ginger, and stir-fry for 30 seconds or until fragrant.
4. Add beef and stir-fry for 3-4 minutes or until browned and cooked.
5. Add mixed vegetables and stir-fry for 2-3 minutes or until vegetables are tender-crisp.
6. Pour the sauce over the beef and vegetables, and stir-fry for another minute or until the sauce thickens and coats the meat and vegetables.
7. Serve hot with cooked brown rice.

Nutritional Values: Calories: 425 Fat: 13g Saturated Fat: 3g Cholesterol: 69mg Sodium: 382mg Carbohydrates: 48g Fiber: 5g Sugars: 8g Protein: 30g

Greek Turkey Burgers

Preparation time: 15 minutes **Cooking Time:** 20 minutes **Servings:** 4

Ingredients:

- For the burgers:
- 1 lb. lean ground turkey
- 1/2 cup crumbled feta cheese
- 1/4 cup chopped fresh parsley.
- 1/4 cup chopped red onion.
- 1 clove garlic, minced.
- 1 tsp dried oregano
- Salt and pepper, to taste
- 4 whole-wheat hamburger buns
- For the sweet potato fries:
- 2 large, sweet potatoes, cut into fries.
- 1 tbsp olive oil
- Salt and pepper, to taste

Instructions:

1. Preheat the oven to 400°F.
2. Mix the ground turkey, feta cheese, parsley, red onion, garlic, oregano, salt, and pepper in a large bowl.
3. Form the mixture into four patties.
4. Heat a grill pan over medium-high heat. Grill the burgers for 5-6 minutes per side or until cooked through.
5. Meanwhile, toss the sweet potato fries with olive oil, salt, and pepper. Arrange in a single layer on a baking sheet and bake for 20-25 minutes or until crispy and tender.
6. Serve the burgers on whole-wheat buns with sweet potato fries on the side.

Nutritional Values: Calories: 430 Fat: 15g Saturated Fat: 5g Cholesterol: 104mg Sodium: 598mg Carbohydrates: 39g Fiber: 6g Sugar: 8g Protein: 35g

Spicy Turkey Chili

Preparation time: 10 minutes **Cooking Time:** 30 minutes **Servings:** 6

Ingredients:

- 1-pound ground turkey
- 1 tablespoon olive oil
- 1 onion, chopped.
- 3 cloves garlic, minced.
- 2 bell peppers, chopped.
- 2 tablespoons chili powder
- 1 teaspoon ground cumin
- 1/4 teaspoon cayenne pepper
- 1 can (28 ounces) crushed tomatoes
- 1 can (15 ounces) of kidney beans, drained and rinsed.
- 1 can (15 ounces) of black beans, drained and rinsed.
- 1/2 cup water
- Salt and black pepper, to taste
- 3 cups cooked brown rice.
- 1 avocado, sliced.

Instructions:

1. In a large pot, heat the olive oil over medium heat. Add the ground turkey and cook until browned, breaking it up with a wooden spoon as it cooks.
2. Add the onion, garlic, and bell peppers to the pot and cook until the vegetables are softened.
3. Add the chili powder, cumin, and cayenne pepper to the pot and combine.
4. Add the crushed tomatoes, kidney beans, black beans, and water to the pot and stir to combine.
5. Bring the chili to a simmer and let it cook for about 20-25 minutes, stirring occasionally.
6. Season the chili with salt and black pepper to taste.
7. To serve, spoon the chili over cooked brown rice and top with sliced avocado.

Nutritional Values: Calories: 395 kcal Protein: 23 g Fat: 15 g Carbohydrates: 48 g Fiber: 14 g Sodium: 501 mg

Beef and Vegetable Kebabs

Preparation time: 20 minutes **Cooking Time:** 15 minutes **Servings:** 4

Ingredients:

- 1-pound beef sirloin, cut into 1-inch cubes.
- 1 red bell pepper, seeded and cut into 1-inch pieces.
- 1 yellow bell pepper, seeded and cut into 1-inch pieces.
- 1 zucchini, sliced into rounds.
- 1 red onion, cut into 1-inch pieces.
- 2 tablespoons olive oil
- 2 tablespoons balsamic vinegar
- 1 teaspoon dried oregano
- Salt and pepper, to taste
- 1 cup brown rice
- 2 cups water

Instructions:

1. Preheat the grill to medium-high heat.
2. Thread beef and vegetables onto skewers, alternating between each one.
3. Whisk together olive oil, balsamic vinegar, dried oregano, salt, and pepper in a small bowl.
4. Brush the kebabs with the olive oil mixture.
5. Place the kebabs on the grill and cook for 10-12 minutes, occasionally turning, until the beef is cooked to your liking and the vegetables are tender.
6. While the kebabs cook, prepare the brown rice according to the instructions.
7. Serve the kebabs with brown rice on the side.

Nutritional Values: Calories: 425 Total Fat: 14g Saturated Fat: 3.5g Cholesterol: 70mg Sodium: 90mg Total Carbohydrates: 43g Dietary Fiber: 5g Sugar: 6g Protein: 33g

Baked Turkey Breast

Preparation time: 10 minutes **Cooking Time:** 40-50 minutes **Servings:** 4

Ingredients:

- 1-pound boneless, skinless turkey breast
- 1 red bell pepper, seeded and sliced into strips.
- 1 yellow bell pepper, seeded and sliced into strips.
- 1 zucchini, sliced into rounds.
- 1 onion, sliced into wedges.
- 2 tablespoons olive oil
- 1 teaspoon dried oregano
- 1/2 teaspoon garlic powder
- Salt and pepper, to taste
- 1 cup quinoa, cooked according to package directions.

Instructions:

1. Preheat the oven to 375°F.
2. In a large baking dish, place the turkey breast in the center and surround it with bell peppers, zucchini, and onion.
3. Drizzle the olive oil over the vegetables and turkey breast, then sprinkle with oregano, garlic powder, salt, and pepper.
4. Bake for 40-50 minutes until the turkey is cooked and the vegetables are tender.
5. Serve with a side of cooked quinoa.

Nutritional Values: Calories: 345 kcal Fat: 10 g Carbohydrates: 29 g Fiber: 5 g Protein: 36 g Sodium: 85 mg

Beef and Broccoli Stir-Fry

Preparation time: 15 minutes **Cooking Time:** 20 minutes **Servings:** 4

Ingredients:

- 1 lb. flank steak, sliced into thin strips.
- 1 head broccoli, cut into florets.
- 1 red bell pepper, sliced into thin strips.
- 1 onion, sliced.
- 2 cloves garlic, minced.
- 1 tbsp. cornstarch

- 1/4 cup low-sodium soy sauce
- 1/4 cup low-sodium beef broth
- 1 tbsp. honey
- 1 tsp sesame oil
- 2 tbsp. vegetable oil
- Salt and pepper, to taste
- 4 cups cooked brown rice.

Instructions:
1. Preheat the oven to 425°F.
2. Whisk together the cornstarch, soy sauce, beef broth, honey, and sesame oil in a small bowl. Set aside.
3. In a large skillet over medium-high heat, add the vegetable oil. When hot, add the sliced steak and cook for 2-3 minutes on each side until browned.
4. Add the broccoli, bell pepper, onion, and garlic to the skillet and cook for another 2-3 minutes, until the vegetables are slightly softened.
5. Pour the sauce over the steak and vegetables and stir well to combine.
6. Transfer the skillet to the oven and bake for 10-12 minutes, until the sauce is bubbly, and the vegetables are tender.
7. Serve the beef and broccoli stir-fry over cooked brown rice.

Nutritional Values: Calories: 421 kcal Fat: 14 g Carbohydrates: 42 g Fiber: 6 g Protein: 33 g Sodium: 599 mg

Pork Tenderloin

Preparation time: 15 minutes **Cooking Time:** 45 minutes **Servings:** 4

Ingredients:
- 1 lb. pork tenderloin, trimmed of excess fat.
- 1 tsp dried thyme
- 1 tsp dried rosemary
- 1 tsp garlic powder
- Salt and pepper to taste
- 1 lb. mixed vegetables (such as carrots, Brussels sprouts, and bell peppers), chopped.
- 1 tbsp. olive oil
- 2 cups cooked brown rice.
- 1 tbsp. chopped fresh parsley.

Instructions:
1. Preheat the oven to 400°F.
2. Combine the thyme, rosemary, garlic powder, salt, and pepper in a small bowl. Rub the spice mixture all over the pork tenderloin.
3. Toss the mixed vegetables with olive oil in a large bowl and season with salt and pepper.
4. Place the pork tenderloin on a baking sheet lined with parchment paper. Arrange the vegetables around the pork.
5. Bake for 30-40 minutes until the pork is cooked and the vegetables are tender and browned.
6. Let the pork rest for 5 minutes before slicing.
7. Serve the sliced pork with roasted vegetables and brown rice. Garnish with fresh parsley.

Nutritional Values: Calories: 318 kcal Fat: 9 g Carbohydrates: 29 g Fiber: 5 g Protein: 30 g

Snacks

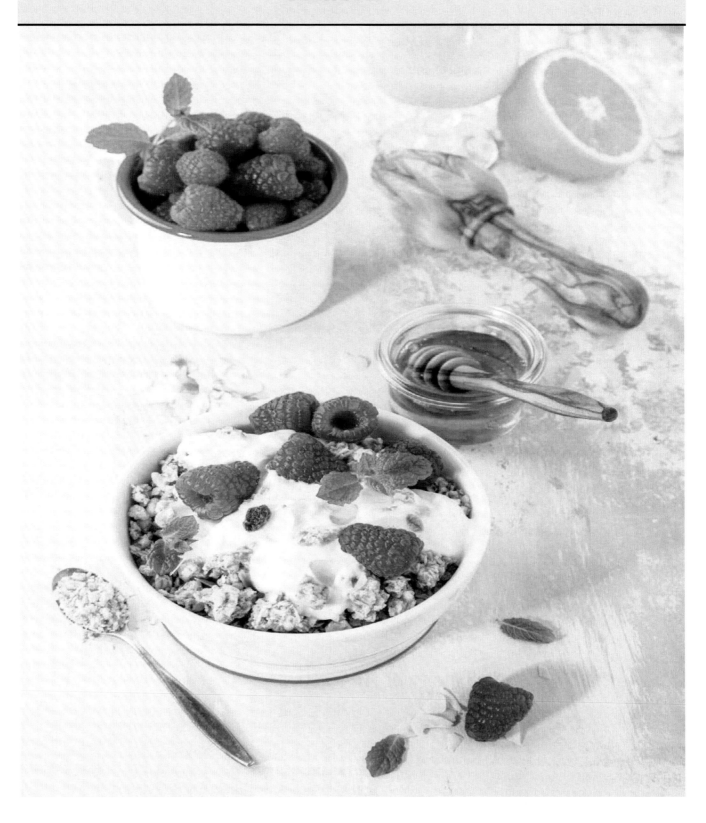

Greek Yogurt with Mixed Berries

Preparation time: 5 minutes. **Servings:** 1
Ingredients:
- 1 cup of nonfat Greek yogurt
- 1/2 cup of mixed berries (such as strawberries, blueberries, and raspberries)
- 1 tablespoon of sliced almonds
- 1 teaspoon of honey (optional)

Instructions:
1. In a small bowl, mix the Greek yogurt and honey (if using).
2. Top the yogurt with mixed berries and sliced almonds.
3. Serve immediately.

Nutritional Values: Calories: 190 kcal Protein: 21 g Fat: 5 g Carbohydrates: 18 g Fiber: 4 g Sodium: 85 mg

Hummus with Whole-Grain Pita Chips

Preparation time: 10 minutes **Cooking Time:** N/A **Servings:** 4
Ingredients:
- 1 can of chickpeas (15 oz.), drained and rinsed.
- 2 garlic cloves, chopped.
- 2 tbsp. tahini
- 3 tbsp. fresh lemon juice
- 2 tbsp. extra-virgin olive oil
- 1/4 tsp ground cumin
- Salt and pepper to taste
- Whole-grain pita chips
- Mixed vegetables, such as carrots, celery, and cucumbers, for dipping

Instructions:
1. In a food processor, blend the chickpeas, garlic, tahini, lemon juice, olive oil, cumin, salt, and pepper until smooth and creamy.
2. Taste and adjust seasoning as necessary.
3. Serve with whole-grain pita chips and mixed vegetables for dipping.

Nutritional Values: Calories: 210 kcal Protein: 8g Fat: 11g Carbohydrates: 22g Fiber: 5g Sodium: 200mg

Trail Mix with Nuts

Ingredients:
- Mixed nuts (unsalted)
- Pumpkin seeds
- Dried cranberries (unsweetened)
- Dried apricots (unsweetened)

Instructions:
1. Measure out desired amounts of each ingredient and mix them in a bowl.
2. Store in an airtight container or portion out into individual snack bags.

Nutritional Values: Calories: 120 Fat: 8g Saturated Fat: 1g Carbohydrates: 9g Fiber: 2g Protein: 4g Sodium: 0mg

Whole-Grain Crackers with Low-Fat Cheese

Preparation time: 10 minutes **Cooking Time:** 15 minutes **Servings:** 4
Ingredients:
- 4 whole-grain crackers
- 1/2 cup low-fat cheese shredded or sliced.
- 1/2 cup grapes, halved.

Instructions:
1. Preheat the oven to 350°F (175°C).
2. Arrange the crackers on a baking sheet.
3. Place a small amount of shredded or sliced cheese on each cracker.
4. Bake for 10-12 minutes or until the cheese is melted and bubbly.
5. Remove from the oven and let cool for a few minutes.
6. Top each cracker with a few halved grapes.
7. Serve and enjoy!

Nutritional Values: Calories: 129 Fat: 5g Carbohydrates: 16g Fiber: 2g Protein: 6g Sodium: 176mg

Roasted Chickpeas with Spices

Preparation time: 5 minutes **Cooking Time:** 35-40 minutes **Servings:** 4
Ingredients:
- 2 cans chickpeas, drained and rinsed.
- 2 tablespoons olive oil
- 1 teaspoon garlic powder

- 1 teaspoon ground cumin
- 1/2 teaspoon smoked paprika.
- Salt and pepper to taste

Instructions:

1. Preheat the oven to 400°F.
2. Toss the chickpeas, olive oil, garlic powder, cumin, smoked paprika, salt, and pepper in a large bowl until evenly coated.
3. Spread the chickpeas in a single layer on a baking sheet.
4. Bake for 35-40 minutes or until crispy, stirring occasionally.
5. Remove from the oven and let cool slightly before serving.

Nutritional Values: Calories: 230 kcal Protein: 10 g Fat: 9 g Carbohydrates: 28 g Fiber: 8 g Sodium: 261 mg

Carrots and Celery Sticks

Preparation time: 10 minutes **Cooking Time:** N/A **Servings:** 4

Ingredients:

- 2 large carrots, peeled and cut into sticks.
- 2 large celery stalks cut into sticks.
- 1/2 cup hummus or guacamole

Instructions:

1. Wash and prepare the carrots and celery by peeling and cutting them into sticks.
2. Place the hummus or guacamole in a small bowl.
3. Arrange the carrot and celery sticks around the bowl of hummus or guacamole.
4. Serve and enjoy as a healthy snack.

Nutritional Values: Calories: 96 kcal Protein: 3 g Fat: 5 g Carbohydrates: 12 g Fiber: 4 g Sodium: 196 mg

Cottage Cheese with Mixed Berries

Preparation time: 5 minutes **Servings:** 1

Ingredients:

- 1/2 cup low-fat cottage cheese
- 1/2 cup mixed berries (blueberries, strawberries, raspberries)

- 1 tablespoon honey

Instructions:

1. Rinse the mixed berries and pat them dry with a paper towel.
2. Spoon the cottage cheese into a bowl.
3. Top the cottage cheese with the mixed berries.
4. Drizzle honey over the top.
5. Serve and enjoy!

Nutritional Values: Calories: 150 kcal Protein: 12g Fat: 2g Carbohydrates: 25g Fiber: 3g Sodium: 330mg

Edamame with Sea Salt

Preparation time: 5 minutes **Cooking Time:** 5-10 minutes **Servings:** 4

Ingredients:

- 2 cups edamame, fresh or frozen
- 1 tsp sea salt

Instructions:

1. If using frozen edamame, thaw them in cold water for a few minutes.
2. In a pot, bring water to a boil and add the edamame.
3. Boil for 5-10 minutes until they are tender.
4. Drain the edamame and transfer them to a serving bowl.
5. Sprinkle sea salt on top of the edamame and toss to coat evenly.
6. Serve warm or cold.

Nutritional Values: Calories: 100 kcal Carbohydrates: 8 g Protein: 10 g Fat: 3 g Sodium: 600 mg Fiber: 4 g

Baked Sweet Potato Chips

Preparation time: 10 minutes **Cooking Time:** 20-25 minutes **Servings:** 4

Ingredients:

- 2 medium sweet potatoes
- 1 tbsp. olive oil
- 1/2 tsp sea salt

Instructions:

1. Preheat oven to 400°F (200°C) and line a baking sheet with parchment paper.

2. Wash the sweet potatoes and slice them into thin rounds using a mandolin or sharp knife.
3. Toss the sweet potato slices with olive oil and sea salt in a large bowl until evenly coated.
4. Arrange the sweet potato slices in a single layer on the prepared baking sheet, ensuring they are not touching.
5. Bake for 20-25 minutes or until the edges are slightly browned, and the chips are crispy.
6. Remove from the oven and let cool for a few minutes before serving.

Nutritional Values: Calories: 90 kcal Fat: 4.5g Carbohydrates: 12g Fiber: 2g Protein: 1g Sodium: 300mg

Roasted Nuts with Cinnamon and Honey

Preparation time: 5 minutes **Cooking Time:** 20-25 minutes **Servings:** 8

Ingredients:
- 2 cups mixed raw nuts (such as almonds, pecans, walnuts, and cashews)
- 1 tablespoon olive oil
- 1 tablespoon honey
- 1 teaspoon cinnamon
- 1/2 teaspoon sea salt

Instructions:
1. Preheat oven to 325°F (165°C).
2. Mix the nuts, olive oil, honey, cinnamon, and salt in a large bowl until the nuts are coated evenly.
3. Spread the mixture onto a baking sheet lined with parchment paper.
4. Roast in the oven for 20-25 minutes or until the nuts are fragrant and lightly toasted, stirring occasionally.
5. Remove from oven and let cool.
6. Store in an airtight container at room temperature for up to two weeks.

Nutritional Values: Calories: 200 kcal Total fat: 18g Saturated fat: 2g Sodium: 75mg Total carbohydrates: 8g Dietary fiber: 3g Sugars: 3g Protein: 6g

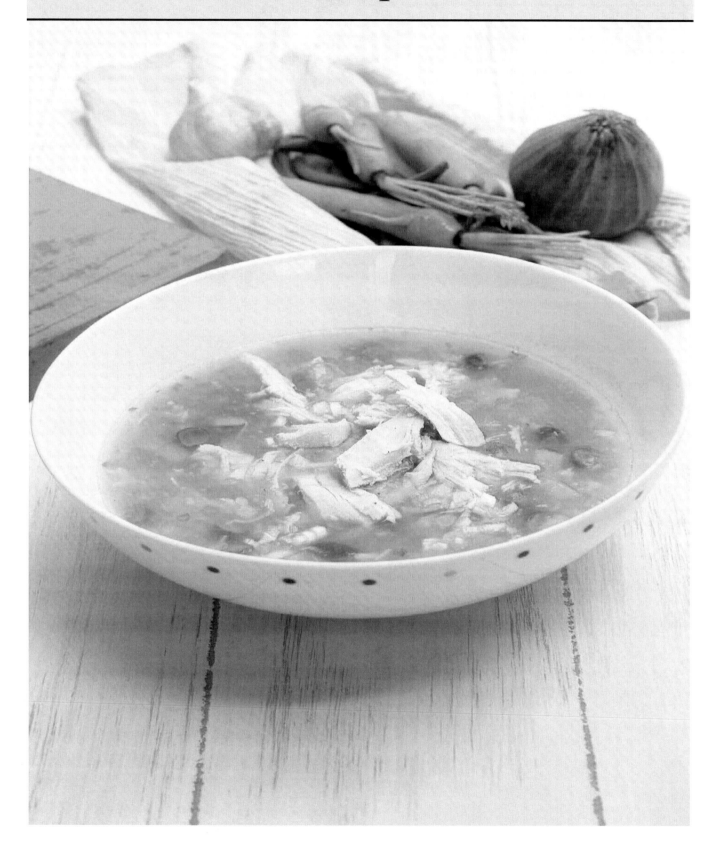

Roasted Tomato and Vegetable Soup

Preparation time: 15 minutes **Cooking Time:** 50 minutes **Servings:** 4

Ingredients:

- 4 large tomatoes, quartered.
- 2 red bell peppers seeded and chopped.
- 1 large onion, chopped.
- 4 cloves garlic, minced.
- 2 cups low-sodium vegetable broth
- 1 tsp dried basil
- 1 tsp dried oregano
- 1 tsp dried thyme
- 1/4 tsp black pepper
- 1/4 tsp sea salt
- 1 tbsp olive oil

Instructions:

1. Preheat oven to 400°F (200°C).
2. Line a baking sheet with parchment paper.
3. Arrange the tomatoes, bell peppers, onion, and garlic on the baking sheet.
4. Drizzle the vegetables with olive oil and sprinkle with salt and black pepper.
5. Roast in the oven for 30-40 minutes or until the vegetables are soft and slightly charred.
6. Transfer the roasted vegetables to a blender or food processor.
7. Add vegetable broth, dried basil, dried oregano, and dried thyme. Blend until smooth.
8. Transfer the blended mixture to a medium saucepan and bring to a boil.
9. Reduce heat to low and let simmer for 5-10 minutes.
10. Serve hot.

Nutritional Values: Calories: 97 kcal Fat: 4g Carbohydrates: 16g Fiber: 4g Protein: 3g Sodium: 209mg

Minestrone Soup with Whole-Grain Bread

Preparation time: 15 minutes **Cooking Time:** 45 minutes **Servings:** 6

Ingredients:

- 1 tablespoon olive oil
- 1 onion, chopped.
- 3 garlic cloves, minced.
- 1 celery stalk, chopped.
- 1 carrot peeled and chopped.
- 1 zucchini, chopped.
- 1 cup green beans, chopped.
- 1 can (28 ounces) diced tomatoes.
- 6 cups low-sodium vegetable broth
- 1 teaspoon dried basil
- 1 teaspoon dried oregano
- 1 teaspoon dried thyme
- 1/2 teaspoon salt
- 1/4 teaspoon black pepper
- 1 can (15 ounces) of kidney beans, rinsed and drained.
- 1 cup whole-wheat macaroni
- 1/4 cup chopped fresh parsley.
- 6 slices whole-grain bread

Instructions:

1. Heat the olive oil in a large pot over medium heat. Add the onion, garlic, celery, carrot, and zucchini, and cook until tender, about 5 minutes.
2. Add the green beans, diced tomatoes, vegetable broth, dried basil, dried oregano, dried thyme, salt, and black pepper to the pot. Bring the soup to a boil, then reduce the heat and simmer for 20 minutes.
3. Add the kidney beans and whole-wheat macaroni to the pot and cook for 10-15 minutes or until the macaroni is tender.
4. Stir in the chopped fresh parsley and serve the soup with whole-grain bread on the side.

Nutritional Values: Calories: 238 kcal Fat: 5 g Carbohydrates: 42 g Fiber: 11 g Protein: 11 g Sodium: 445 mg

Black Bean Soup with Cilantro and Lime

Preparation time: 10 minutes **Cooking Time:** 30 minutes **Servings:** 4

Ingredients:

- 2 cans (15 ounces each) of black beans, rinsed and drained.
- 1 tablespoon olive oil
- 1 onion, chopped.
- 1 red bell pepper, chopped.
- 4 garlic cloves, minced.
- 2 teaspoons ground cumin
- 1 teaspoon chili powder
- 1/2 teaspoon ground coriander
- 1/4 teaspoon cayenne pepper
- 3 cups low-sodium vegetable broth
- 1/4 cup chopped fresh cilantro.
- 2 tablespoons lime juice
- Salt and pepper, to taste

Instructions:

1. Heat the olive oil in a large pot over medium heat. Add the onion and red bell pepper and cook for 5-7 minutes or until softened.
2. Add the garlic, cumin, chili powder, coriander, and cayenne pepper to the pot. Cook for 1-2 minutes, stirring frequently.
3. Add the black beans and vegetable broth to the pot. Bring to a boil, reduce heat, and simmer for 15-20 minutes.
4. Use an immersion blender or transfer the soup to a blender and puree until smooth.
5. Stir in the cilantro and lime juice. Season with salt and pepper to taste.
6. Serve hot.

Nutritional Values: Calories: 215 Fat: 4.8g Saturated Fat: 0.6g Cholesterol: 0mg Carbohydrates: 34.8g Fiber: 11.3g Protein: 11.6g Sodium: 123mg

Greek Lemon Chicken Soup

Preparation time: 15 minutes **Cooking Time:** 45 minutes **Servings:** 6

Ingredients:

- 6 cups low-sodium chicken broth
- 1-pound boneless, skinless chicken breast
- 1 cup brown rice, uncooked
- 2 cups chopped spinach.
- 1/2 cup chopped onion.
- 2 garlic cloves, minced.
- 1/4 cup lemon juice
- 1 teaspoon lemon zest
- 1 teaspoon dried oregano
- Salt and pepper, to taste
- 2 large eggs
- 1/4 cup chopped fresh parsley.

Instructions:

1. In a large pot, bring the chicken broth to a boil. Add the chicken breasts and reduce heat to low. Simmer for 20 minutes or until chicken is cooked through.
2. Remove chicken breasts from the pot and set aside to cool. Once cool, shred the chicken into bite-sized pieces.
3. Add the rice, spinach, onion, garlic, lemon juice, lemon zest, oregano, salt, and pepper to the pot. Stir to combine.
4. Increase heat to medium-high and bring the soup to a boil. Reduce heat to low and let simmer for 20-25 minutes or until rice is cooked.
5. In a small bowl, whisk together the eggs and parsley. Slowly pour the egg mixture into the soup while stirring gently. Continue for 1-2 minutes or until the egg is cooked.
6. Serve hot with additional lemon wedges and fresh parsley, if desired.

Nutritional Values: Calories: 249kcal Fat: 4g Saturated Fat: 1g Cholesterol: 87mg Sodium: 260mg Potassium: 609mg Carbohydrates: 27g Fiber: 2g Sugar: 2g Protein: 26g

Sweet Potato and Black Bean Soup

Preparation time: 15 minutes **Cooking Time:** 30 minutes **Servings:** 4

Ingredients:

- 2 large, sweet potatoes, peeled and diced.
- 1 tablespoon olive oil
- 1 large onion, chopped.
- 2 cloves garlic, minced.
- 1 teaspoon cumin
- 1 teaspoon chili powder
- 1/2 teaspoon paprika
- 1 can (15 ounces) of black beans, drained and rinsed.
- 1 can (14.5 ounces) diced tomatoes.
- 4 cups low-sodium vegetable broth
- Salt and pepper to taste
- Optional toppings: chopped cilantro, sour cream, diced avocado

Instructions:

1. Heat the olive oil over medium heat in a large pot or Dutch oven. Add the onion and garlic and cook until the onion is softened and translucent, about 5 minutes.
2. Add the sweet potatoes and spices to the pot and stir to combine. Cook for 2-3 minutes, stirring occasionally.
3. Add the black beans, diced tomatoes, and vegetable broth to the pot. Stir to combine.
4. Bring the mixture to a boil, then reduce the heat and simmer for 20-25 minutes or until the sweet potatoes are tender.
5. Use an immersion blender to puree the soup until it is smooth, leaving some chunks for texture.
6. Taste the soup and season with salt and pepper as needed.
7. Serve hot, garnished with chopped cilantro, a dollop of sour cream, and/or diced avocado, if desired.

Nutritional Values: Calories: 236 Total fat: 5g Saturated fat: 1g Cholesterol: 0mg Sodium: 472mg Total carbohydrate: 43g Dietary fiber: 11g Total sugars: 10g Protein: 8g

Chicken and Vegetable Noodle Soup

Preparation time: 20 minutes **Cooking Time:** 25 minutes **Servings:** 6

Ingredients:

- 1 tablespoon olive oil
- 1 onion, chopped.
- 2 cloves garlic, minced.
- 2 celery stalks, chopped.
- 2 carrots peeled and chopped.
- 1 red bell pepper seeded and chopped.
- 6 cups low-sodium chicken broth
- 2 cups water
- 1 teaspoon dried thyme
- 1 teaspoon dried oregano
- 1/2 teaspoon salt
- 1/4 teaspoon black pepper
- 1-pound boneless, skinless chicken breasts cut into bite-sized pieces
- 2 cups uncooked whole-grain noodles
- 2 tablespoons chopped fresh parsley.

Instructions:

1. Heat the olive oil in a large pot or Dutch oven over medium heat.
2. Add the onion, garlic, and sauté until tender, about 3-4 minutes.
3. Add the celery, carrots, and bell pepper and continue to sauté for another 5 minutes.
4. Add the chicken broth, water, thyme, oregano, salt, and black pepper to the pot and boil.
5. Reduce the heat to low and add the chicken and noodles. Simmer until the chicken is cooked and the noodles are tender about 10-12 minutes.
6. Stir in the chopped parsley and serve hot.

Nutritional Values: Calories: 240 kcal Fat: 5 g Saturated Fat: 1 g Carbohydrates: 24 g Fiber: 4 g Protein: 24 g Sodium: 310 mg

Butternut Squash Soup with Apple and Ginger

Preparation time: 20 minutes **Cooking Time:** 40 minutes **Servings:** 4

Ingredients:

- 1 butternut squash, peeled and cubed (about 4 cups)
- 1 large apple peeled and chopped.
- 1 onion, chopped.
- 2 cloves garlic, minced.
- 2 teaspoons grated ginger
- 4 cups low-sodium chicken or vegetable broth
- 1/2 cup unsweetened almond milk
- 1/2 teaspoon ground cinnamon
- 1/4 teaspoon ground nutmeg
- Salt and pepper to taste
- 1 tablespoon olive oil

Instructions:

1. Heat the olive oil over medium heat in a large pot or Dutch oven.
2. Add the onion and cook until translucent, about 5 minutes.
3. Add the garlic and ginger and cook for another 1-2 minutes.
4. Add the butternut squash, apple, broth, cinnamon, nutmeg, salt, and pepper. Stir to combine.
5. Bring the soup to a boil, then reduce the heat and let it simmer for about 20-25 minutes until the vegetables are tender.
6. Remove the soup from the heat.
7. Using an immersion blender or a blender, puree the soup until smooth.
8. Return the soup to the pot and stir in the almond milk.
9. Heat the soup over low heat until warmed through.
10. Serve hot, garnished with a sprinkle of cinnamon and some chopped fresh herbs, if desired.

Nutritional Values: Calories: 160 kcal Fat: 4.5 g Carbohydrates: 29 g Fiber: 6 g Protein: 4 g Sodium: 130 mg

Vegetable and Quinoa Soup

Preparation time: 15 minutes **Cooking Time:** 30 minutes **Servings:** 6

Ingredients:

- 1 tablespoon olive oil
- 1 onion, chopped.
- 2 cloves garlic, minced.
- 2 carrots peeled and chopped.
- 2 stalks of celery, chopped.
- 1 red bell pepper, chopped.
- 1 zucchini, chopped.
- 1 yellow squash, chopped.
- 1 can (14.5 ounces) diced tomatoes, undrained.
- 6 cups low-sodium vegetable broth
- 1/2 cup uncooked quinoa rinsed and drained.
- 2 teaspoons dried thyme
- 2 teaspoons dried rosemary
- 1/4 cup chopped fresh parsley.
- 1/4 cup chopped fresh basil.
- Salt and pepper to taste

Instructions:

1. In a large pot, heat the olive oil over medium heat. Add the onion and garlic and cook until the onion is translucent, and the garlic is fragrant about 3 minutes.
2. Add the carrots, celery, red bell pepper, zucchini, and yellow squash to the pot. Cook, stirring occasionally, until the vegetables are slightly tender, about 5 minutes.
3. Add the diced tomatoes (with their juice), vegetable broth, quinoa, thyme, and rosemary to the pot. Stir to combine.
4. Bring the soup to a boil, then reduce the heat to low and simmer for 20-25 minutes or until the vegetables and quinoa are tender.
5. Stir in the parsley and basil. Season with salt and pepper to taste.
6. Serve hot, garnished with additional fresh herbs if desired.

Nutritional Values: Calories: 141kcal Fat: 3g Carbohydrates: 24g Fiber: 5g Protein: 6g Sodium: 118mg

Broccoli and Cheddar Soup

Preparation time: 10 minutes **Cooking Time:** 30 minutes **Servings:** 4

Ingredients:

- 2 tablespoons olive oil
- 1 onion, chopped.
- 3 cloves garlic, minced.
- 4 cups broccoli florets
- 4 cups low-sodium vegetable broth
- 1 cup unsweetened almond milk
- 1 cup shredded low-fat cheddar cheese.
- Salt and pepper to taste
- Whole-grain crackers for serving.

Instructions:

1. Heat the olive oil in a large pot over medium heat. Add the onion, garlic, and sauté until the onion is translucent, about 5 minutes.
2. Add the broccoli florets and vegetable broth to the pot. Bring to a boil, then reduce heat and simmer until the broccoli is tender, about 20 minutes.
3. Remove the pot from heat and let cool for a few minutes. Then, using an immersion blender or transfer to a blender, blend the soup until smooth.
4. Return the soup to the pot and stir in the almond milk and cheddar cheese until the cheese is melted and the soup is well combined.
5. Season with salt and pepper to taste.
6. Serve hot with whole-grain crackers on the side.

Nutritional Values: Calories: 204 Fat: 12g Saturated Fat: 3.3g Cholesterol: 12mg Sodium: 256mg Carbohydrates: 18g Fiber: 4g Sugar: 6g Protein: 11g

Creamy Tomato and Basil Soup

Preparation time: 10 minutes **Cooking Time:** 30 minutes **Servings:** 4

Ingredients:

- 1 tablespoon olive oil
- 1 small onion, chopped.
- 2 cloves garlic, minced.
- 28 oz can crush tomatoes.
- 1 cup low-sodium vegetable broth
- 1/2 cup fat-free half and half
- 1/4 cup chopped fresh basil.
- Salt and black pepper to taste
- 4 slices of whole-grain bread, toasted.

Instructions:

1. Heat the olive oil in a large pot over medium heat.
2. Add the chopped onion and cook until softened about 5 minutes.
3. Add the minced garlic and cook for another minute.
4. Add the crushed tomatoes and vegetable broth to the pot and stir well.
5. Bring the mixture to a boil, then reduce heat to low and simmer for 20 minutes.
6. Use an immersion blender or transfer the soup to a blender and puree until smooth.
7. Stir in the half and half and chopped basil and heat through.
8. Season with salt and black pepper to taste.
9. Serve hot with toasted whole-grain bread on the side.

Nutritional Values: Calories: 170 kcal Fat: 5 g Sodium: 370 mg Carbohydrates: 27 g Fiber: 5 g Protein: 6 g

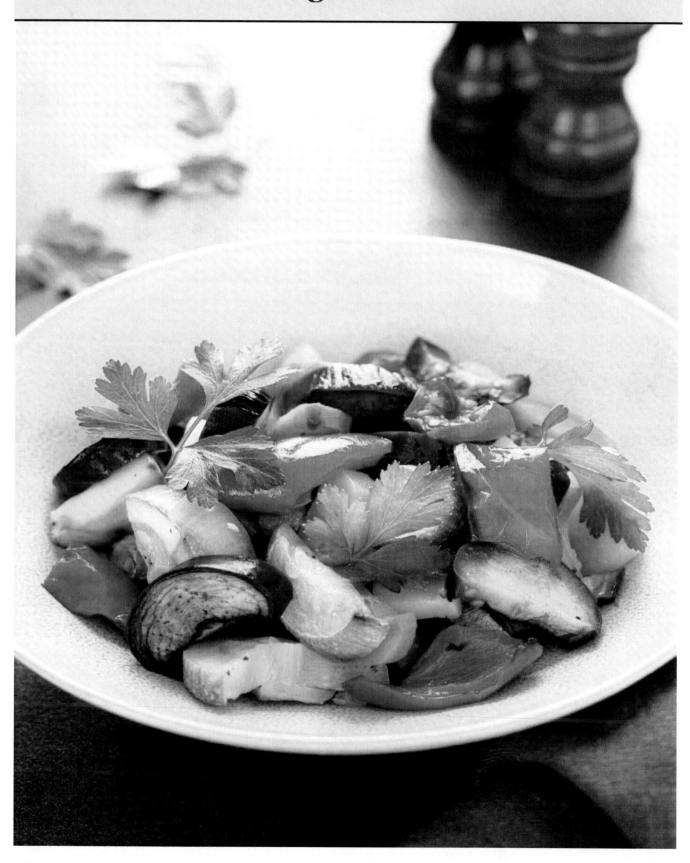

Roasted Asparagus with Lemon and Garlic

Preparation time: 5 minutes Cooking **Time:** 15 minutes Servings: 4

Ingredients:

- 1-pound fresh asparagus, trimmed
- 2 tablespoons olive oil
- 2 cloves garlic, minced.
- 1 lemon juiced and zested.
- Salt and pepper to taste

Instructions:

1. Preheat the oven to 400°F (200°C).
2. Arrange the asparagus in a single layer on a baking sheet.
3. Drizzle the olive oil over the asparagus and toss to coat evenly.
4. Sprinkle the garlic, lemon zest, and lemon juice over the asparagus and toss to coat.
5. Season with salt and pepper to taste.
6. Roast in the oven for 12-15 minutes or until the asparagus is tender but slightly crisp.
7. Serve hot as a side dish.

Nutritional Values: Calories: 76 kcal Fat: 7g Carbohydrates: 4g Fiber: 2g Protein: 2g Sodium: 2mg

Garlic and Herb Roasted Mushrooms

Preparation time: 10 minutes **Cooking Time:** 20 minutes **Servings:** 4

Ingredients:

- 16 oz. mushrooms cleaned and sliced.
- 2 tbsp. olive oil
- 2 garlic cloves, minced.
- 1 tbsp. fresh thyme leaves
- 1 tbsp. fresh rosemary leaves
- Salt and black pepper, to taste

Instructions:

1. Preheat the oven to 400°F.
2. Mix the olive oil, minced garlic, thyme, rosemary, salt, and black pepper in a bowl.
3. Add the sliced mushrooms and toss to coat.

4. Arrange the mushrooms in a single layer on a baking sheet.
5. Roast in the oven for 20 minutes or until the mushrooms are tender and golden brown.
6. Remove from the oven and serve hot.

Nutritional Values: Calories: 90 kcal Fat: 7 g Carbohydrates: 5 g Fiber: 1 g Protein: 3 g Sodium: 152 mg

Sautéed Green Beans with Toasted Almonds

Preparation time: 10 minutes **Cooking Time:** 15 minutes **Servings:** 4

Ingredients:

- 1 lb. green beans, trimmed.
- 2 tbsp. olive oil
- 2 cloves garlic, minced.
- 1/4 cup slivered almonds
- Salt and pepper, to taste

Instructions:

1. Heat the olive oil in a large skillet over medium heat.
2. Add the green beans to the skillet and sauté for 5-7 minutes or until they soften.
3. Add the garlic to the skillet and sauté for 1-2 minutes or until fragrant.
4. Add the slivered almonds to the skillet and sauté for 2-3 minutes, until they are toasted and golden brown.
5. Season with salt and pepper to taste.
6. Serve hot and enjoy!

Nutritional Values: Calories: 110 kcal Fat: 9 g Carbohydrates: 7 g Protein: 2 g Sodium: 150 mg Fiber: 3 g

Steamed Broccoli

Preparation time: 5 minutes **Cooking Time:** 10 minutes **Servings:** 4

Ingredients:

- 1-pound broccoli florets
- 2 garlic cloves, minced.
- 1 lemon juiced and zested.
- 2 tablespoons olive oil
- Salt and pepper, to taste

Instructions:

1. Rinse the broccoli florets under running water and place them in a steamer basket.
2. Add water to a pot and bring it to a boil. Once boiling, place the steamer basket with the broccoli over the pool and cover it with a lid.
3. Steam the broccoli for about 8-10 minutes or until tender but still crisp.
4. While the broccoli is steaming, heat the olive oil in a pan over medium heat.
5. Add the minced garlic to the pan and sauté for 1-2 minutes or until fragrant.
6. Remove the pan from the heat and add the lemon juice and zest to the pan. Mix well.
7. Once the broccoli is steamed, transfer it to a large bowl and pour the lemon-garlic mixture over the top.
8. Toss the broccoli until it is well coated with the mixture.
9. Season with salt and pepper to taste.
10. Serve warm.

Nutritional Values: Calories: 84 kcal Fat: 6.7 g Carbohydrates: 7.4 g Fiber: 2.9 g Protein: 3.3 g Sodium: 36 mg

Balsamic Roasted Carrots

Preparation time: 10 minutes **Cooking Time:** 25 minutes **Servings:** 4
Ingredients:

- 1-pound carrots, peeled and sliced into 1-inch pieces
- 1 tablespoon olive oil
- 1 tablespoon balsamic vinegar
- 2 cloves garlic, minced.
- 1 teaspoon dried thyme
- 1 teaspoon dried rosemary
- 1/2 teaspoon salt
- 1/4 teaspoon black pepper

Instructions:

1. Preheat the oven to 400°F (200°C).
2. Mix the olive oil, balsamic vinegar, garlic, thyme, rosemary, salt, and black pepper in a large bowl.
3. Add the sliced carrots to the bowl and toss to coat with the herb mixture.
4. Spread the carrots in a single layer on a baking sheet lined with parchment paper.
5. Roast the carrots for 20-25 minutes or until tender and lightly browned.
6. Serve hot as a side dish.

Nutritional Values: Calories: 85kcal Fat: 4g Carbohydrates: 13g Fiber: 4g Protein: 1g Sodium: 350mg

Garlic Roasted Cherry Tomatoes

Preparation time: 5 minutes **Cooking Time:** 15-20 minutes **Servings:** 4
Ingredients:

- 2 cups cherry tomatoes
- 2 garlic cloves, minced.
- 1 tablespoon olive oil
- 1/4 teaspoon salt
- 1/8 teaspoon black pepper
- 1 tablespoon chopped fresh basil.

Instructions:

1. Preheat the oven to 400°F (200°C).
2. Mix the minced garlic, olive oil, salt, and black pepper in a small bowl.
3. Place the cherry tomatoes in a baking dish, drizzle the garlic and oil mixture over them, and toss to coat.
4. Roast the cherry tomatoes for 15-20 minutes until they wrinkle and burst.
5. Remove from the oven and sprinkle with chopped fresh basil before serving.

Nutritional Values: Calories: 48kcal Fat: 3g Saturated Fat: 0g Cholesterol: 0mg Sodium: 150mg Potassium: 206mg Carbohydrates: 4g Fiber: 1g Sugar: 2g Protein: 1g

Grilled Eggplant with Balsamic Glaze

Preparation time: 10 minutes **Cooking Time:** 10 minutes **Servings:** 4
Ingredients:

- 2 medium eggplants, sliced into rounds.
- 1/4 cup balsamic vinegar
- 2 tablespoons olive oil

- 2 garlic cloves, minced.
- Salt and pepper, to taste
- 1/4 cup fresh parsley, chopped.

Instructions:

1. Preheat the grill to medium-high heat.
2. Whisk together balsamic vinegar, olive oil, garlic, salt, and pepper in a small bowl.
3. Brush both sides of the eggplant slices with the balsamic mixture.
4. Place eggplant slices on the grill and cook for 4-5 minutes per side or until tender and slightly charred.
5. Remove eggplant from the grill and sprinkle with fresh parsley.
6. Serve immediately.

Nutritional Values: Calories: 109 Fat: 7g Protein: 2g Carbohydrates: 12g Fiber: 6g Sodium: 6mg

Spicy Roasted Cauliflower

Preparation time: 10 minutes **Cooking Time:** 20 minutes **Servings:** 4

Ingredients:

- 1 large head of cauliflower, cut into bite-sized florets.
- 2 tbsp olive oil
- 3 cloves garlic, minced.
- 1 tsp dried oregano
- 1/2 tsp dried thyme
- 1/2 tsp smoked paprika.
- 1/4 tsp cayenne pepper (adjust to taste)
- Salt and pepper, to taste
- Fresh parsley, chopped, for garnish.

Instructions:

1. Preheat the oven to 425°F (220°C).
2. Combine the cauliflower florets, olive oil, minced garlic, oregano, thyme, smoked paprika, cayenne pepper, salt, and pepper in a large bowl. Toss well to coat evenly.
3. Spread the cauliflower mixture in a single layer on a baking sheet.
4. Roast in the oven for 15-20 minutes or until the cauliflower is tender and golden brown.

5. Remove from the oven and let cool for a few minutes. Garnish with chopped fresh parsley before serving.

Nutritional Values: Calories: 92 kcal Fat: 7 g Carbohydrates: 7 g Fiber: 3 g Protein: 3 g Sodium: 17 mg

Roasted Butternut Squash with Maple Syrup

Preparation time: 15 minutes **Cooking Time:** 40 minutes **Servings:** 4

Ingredients:

- 1 medium butternut squash, peeled, seeded, and cubed.
- 1 tablespoon olive oil
- 1 tablespoon maple syrup
- 1 teaspoon ground cinnamon
- Salt and black pepper, to taste

Instructions:

1. Preheat the oven to 400°F (200°C).
2. Mix the butternut squash cubes with olive oil, maple syrup, cinnamon, salt, and black pepper in a bowl.
3. Spread the mixture on a baking sheet and roast in the oven for 40 minutes or until the squash is tender and lightly browned.
4. Serve hot.

Nutritional Values: Calories: 108 kcal Fat: 3 g Carbohydrates: 22 g Fiber: 4 g Protein: 2 g Sodium: 85 mg

Sauteed Spinach with Garlic and Lemon

Preparation time: 5 minutes **Cooking Time:** 5 minutes **Servings:** 4

Ingredients:

- 1 lb. fresh spinach washed and trimmed.
- 2 tbsp. olive oil
- 3 cloves garlic, minced.
- 1/2 tsp salt
- 1/4 tsp black pepper
- Juice of 1 lemon

Instructions:

1. Heat the olive oil in a large skillet over medium heat.

2. Add the minced garlic and sauté for 1-2 minutes until fragrant.
3. Add the spinach to the skillet and toss with the garlic until wilted, about 2-3 minutes.
4. Season with salt and black pepper to taste.
5. Squeeze the juice of 1 lemon over the spinach and toss to combine.
6. Serve hot and enjoy!

Nutritional Values: Calories: 81 kcal Fat: 7 g Carbohydrates: 4 g Protein: 3 g Sodium: 328 mg Potassium: 551 mg Fiber: 2 g Vitamin A: 116% Vitamin C: 45% Calcium: 10% Iron: 18%

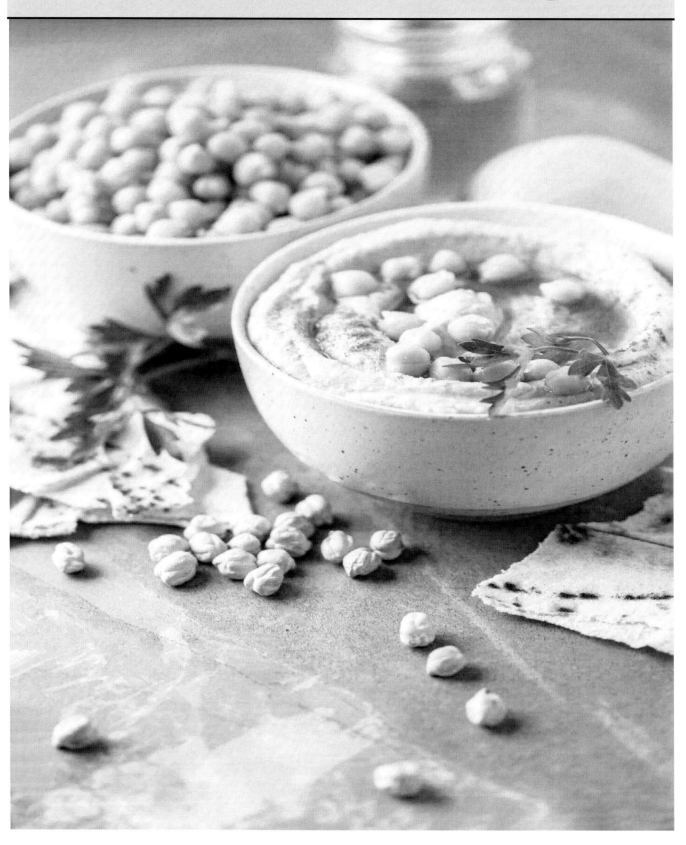

Tomato Sauce with Fresh Herbs

Preparation time: 10 minutes **Cooking Time:** 30 minutes **Servings:** 4

Ingredients:

- 2 tbsp. olive oil
- 1 small onion finely chopped.
- 3 garlic cloves, minced.
- 1 can (28 oz.) crushed tomatoes
- 1 tbsp. tomato paste
- 1/2 tsp salt
- 1/4 tsp black pepper
- 1/4 cup chopped fresh basil.
- 2 tbsp. chopped fresh parsley.
- 1 tbsp. chopped fresh oregano.

Instructions:

1. Heat the olive oil in a large saucepan over medium heat.
2. Add the onion and garlic and cook for 3-4 minutes until softened.
3. Add the crushed tomatoes, tomato paste, salt, and black pepper to the saucepan and stir well.
4. Bring the mixture to a boil, then reduce the heat to low and simmer for 20-25 minutes until the sauce thickens.
5. Add the fresh herbs to the sauce and stir well.
6. Simmer for another 5 minutes, then remove from heat and let cool.
7. Once cooled, use an immersion blender, or transfer the sauce to a blender and blend until smooth.

Nutritional Values: Calories: 100 kcal Fat: 7g Carbohydrates: 8g Fiber: 2g Protein: 2g Sodium: 375mg

Basil Pesto with Almonds

Preparation time: 10 minutes **Servings:** 6

Ingredients:

- 2 cups fresh basil leaves
- 1/2 cup toasted almonds
- 2 cloves garlic, minced.
- 1/4 cup grated Parmesan cheese.
- 1/4 cup olive oil
- Salt and pepper to taste

Instructions:

1. Pulse the basil, almonds, and garlic in a food processor until finely chopped.
2. Add the Parmesan cheese and pulse again until combined.
3. With the food processor running, slowly pour the olive oil until the pesto is smooth and creamy.
4. Season with salt and pepper to taste.

Nutritional Values: Calories: 151 kcal Protein: 4.5 g Carbohydrates: 2.6 g Fat: 14.7 g Saturated Fat: 2.4 g Fiber: 1.6 g Sodium: 95 mg

Greek Yogurt and Cucumber Dip

Preparation time: 10 minutes **Cooking Time:** 0 minutes **Servings:** 6

Ingredients:

- 1 cup Greek yogurt
- 1 cucumber, peeled, seeded, and grated.
- 1 clove garlic, minced.
- 1 tablespoon lemon juice
- 1 tablespoon fresh dill, chopped.
- Salt and pepper to taste

Instructions:

1. Combine Greek yogurt, grated cucumber, minced garlic, lemon juice, and chopped dill in a bowl. Mix well.
2. Season with salt and pepper to taste.
3. Cover and chill in the refrigerator for at least 30 minutes before serving.

4. Serve with fresh vegetables, pita chips, or crackers.

Nutritional Values: Calories: 45 kcal Fat: 1 g Carbohydrates: 4 g Fiber: 0.5 g Protein: 6 g Sodium: 28 mg

Homemade Vegetable Broth

Preparation time: 15 minutes **Cooking Time:** 60 minutes **Servings:** 8 cups
Ingredients:

- 2 onions, chopped.
- 4 cloves garlic, minced.
- 2 carrots, chopped.
- 2 celery stalks, chopped.
- 2 bay leaves
- 8 cups water
- 1/2 teaspoon salt
- 1/4 teaspoon black pepper
- 1/4 teaspoon dried thyme
- 1/4 teaspoon dried oregano

Instructions:

1. Add onions, garlic, carrots, celery, and bay leaves in a large pot. Add water, salt, pepper, thyme, and oregano. Bring to a boil.
2. Reduce heat to low and let the broth simmer for about an hour until the vegetables are soft and the flavors have melded.
3. Remove the bay leaves and strain the broth through a fine-mesh sieve or cheesecloth. Discard the vegetables.
4. Let the broth cool before storing it in an airtight container in the refrigerator or freezer.

Nutritional Values: Calories: 20 Fat: 0g Carbohydrates: 4g Protein: 1g Sodium: 300mg Potassium: 110mg Fiber: 1g

Homemade Salsa with Fresh Tomatoes

Preparation time: 10 minutes **Cooking Time:** N/A **Servings:** 4
Ingredients:

- 4 medium-sized tomatoes, diced.
- 1/2 red onion, diced.
- 1 jalapeño pepper seeded and minced.
- 1/4 cup fresh cilantro, chopped.
- 1 garlic clove, minced.
- 1 tablespoon lime juice
- Salt and pepper, to taste

Instructions:

1. Combine diced tomatoes, red onion, jalapeño pepper, cilantro, and minced garlic in a medium-sized bowl.
2. Add lime juice to the bowl and stir well to combine.
3. Season with salt and pepper to taste.
4. Refrigerate for at least 30 minutes before serving to allow the flavors to meld together.

Nutritional Values: Calories: 30 kcal Fat: 0.3 g Carbohydrates: 6 g Fiber: 1.7 g Protein: 1.5 g Sodium: 10 mg

Homemade Hummus with Chickpeas

Preparation time: 10 minutes **Cooking Time:** 0 minutes **Servings:** 6
Ingredients:

- 1 can (15 oz.) chickpeas, drained and rinsed.
- 1/4 cup tahini
- 2 cloves garlic, minced.
- 2 tablespoons lemon juice
- 1/2 teaspoon ground cumin
- 1/2 teaspoon salt
- 2 tablespoons water
- Optional: paprika, chopped parsley, and/or extra-virgin olive oil for garnish

Instructions:

1. Combine chickpeas, tahini, garlic, lemon juice, cumin, salt, and water in a food processor or blender. Blend until smooth and creamy, adding more water to achieve desired consistency.
2. Taste and adjust seasoning as needed.
3. Transfer hummus to a serving bowl and garnish with paprika, chopped parsley, and/or a drizzle of extra-virgin olive oil, if desired.
4. Serve with fresh vegetables, whole-grain pita bread, or crackers.

Nutritional Values: Calories: 118 kcal Fat: 7 g Carbohydrates: 11 g Fiber: 3 g Protein: 4 g Sodium: 222 mg

BBQ Sauce with Fresh Ingredients

Preparation time: 10 minutes **Cooking Time:** 15 minutes **Servings:** 8
Ingredients:

- 1/2 cup chopped onion.
- 3 cloves garlic, minced.
- 1 cup ketchup
- 1/2 cup apple cider vinegar
- 1/4 cup honey
- 2 tablespoons Dijon mustard
- 2 tablespoons Worcestershire sauce
- 1 tablespoon paprika
- 1/4 teaspoon cayenne pepper
- Salt and pepper, to taste

Instructions:

1. In a medium saucepan over medium heat, sauté the onion until soft and translucent, about 5 minutes. Add the garlic and cook for an additional 1-2 minutes.
2. Add the ketchup, apple cider vinegar, honey, Dijon mustard, Worcestershire

sauce, paprika, and cayenne pepper to the saucepan. Whisk until combined.
3. Bring the mixture to a simmer and cook for 10-15 minutes, stirring occasionally, until the sauce has thickened slightly.
4. Season with salt and pepper to taste.
5. Remove the sauce from heat and let it cool before storing it in an airtight container in the refrigerator for up to 1 week.

Nutritional Values: Calories: 70 Fat: 0.2 g Saturated Fat: 0 g Cholesterol: 0 mg Carbohydrates: 18 g Fiber: 0.4 g Sugar: 15 g Protein: 0.6 g Sodium: 274 mg

Garlic and Herb Marinade for Chicken

Preparation time: 10 minutes. **Servings:** 4
Ingredients:

- 4 cloves garlic, minced.
- 2 tablespoons fresh parsley, chopped.
- 1 tablespoon fresh thyme, chopped.
- 1 tablespoon fresh rosemary, chopped.
- 1/4 cup olive oil
- 2 tablespoons lemon juice
- Salt and pepper to taste

Instructions:

1. Mix the minced garlic, chopped parsley, thyme, and rosemary in a small bowl.
2. Add in the olive oil and lemon juice and mix well.
3. Season with salt and pepper to taste.
4. Place your chicken or fish in a resealable plastic bag or shallow dish.
5. Pour the marinade over the chicken or fish, ensuring it is fully coated.
6. Cover the dish or seal the bag and marinate in the refrigerator for at least 30 minutes or up to 8 hours for maximum flavor.

7. When ready to cook, remove the chicken or fish from the marinade and discard any excess marinade.

8. Grill, bake or pan-sear the chicken or fish until cooked through.

Nutritional Values: Calories: 147 kcal Fat: 14.8 g Carbohydrates: 2.7 g Protein: 1.1 g Sodium: 148 mg
Potassium: 45 mg Fiber: 0.4 g

Homemade Ranch Dressing with Greek Yogurt

Preparation time: 10 minutes. **Servings:** 8

Ingredients:

- 1 cup plain Greek yogurt.
- 1/4 cup of low-fat milk
- 1 tablespoon dried dill weed.
- 1 tablespoon dried parsley
- 1 tablespoon dried chives
- 1/2 teaspoon garlic powder
- 1/2 teaspoon onion powder
- 1/4 teaspoon salt
- 1/8 teaspoon black pepper

Instructions:

1. Whisk together the Greek yogurt and milk in a small bowl until smooth.
2. Stir in the dill weed, parsley, chives, garlic powder, onion powder, salt, and black pepper until well combined.
3. Taste and adjust seasoning as needed.
4. Refrigerate until ready to use

Nutritional Values: Calories: 24 kcal Fat: 1 g Carbohydrates: 2 g Protein: 3 g Sodium: 78 mg

Lemon and Herb Vinaigrette

Preparation time: 5 minutes. **Servings:** 6

Ingredients:

- 1/4 cup freshly squeezed lemon juice.

- 1/4 cup extra-virgin olive oil
- 1 tablespoon Dijon mustard
- 1 tablespoon honey
- 1 garlic clove, minced.
- 1 teaspoon dried oregano
- 1 teaspoon dried thyme
- Salt and black pepper to taste

Instructions:

1. In a small bowl, whisk together lemon juice, olive oil, Dijon mustard, honey, minced garlic, dried oregano, dried thyme, salt, and black pepper until well combined.
2. Taste and adjust seasonings, if necessary.
3. Serve immediately or refrigerate until ready to use.

Nutritional Values: Calories: 91kcal Fat: 9g Saturated Fat: 1g Sodium: 60mg Carbohydrates: 3g Fiber: 0g Sugar: 3g Protein: 0g

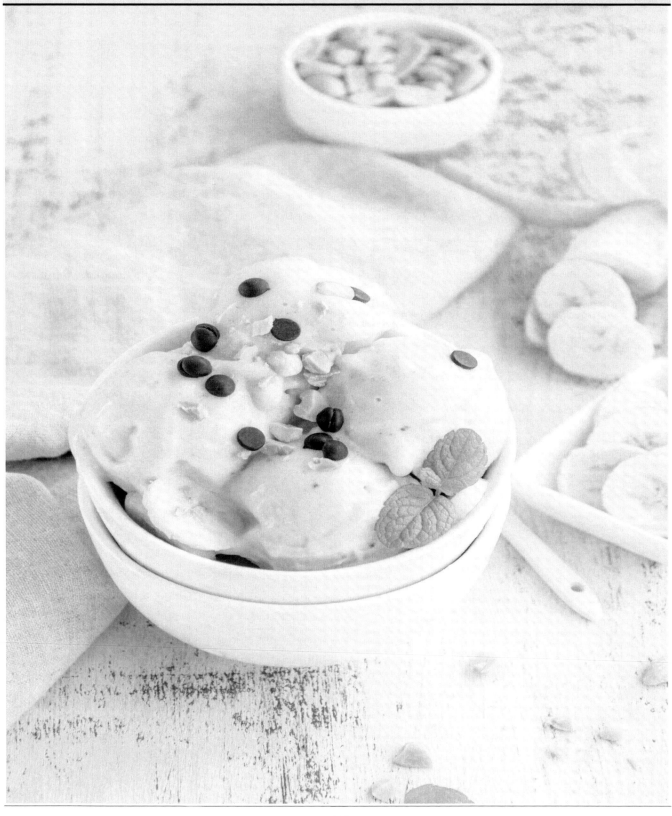

Fresh Fruit Salad with Greek Yogurt and Honey

Preparation time: 15 minutes. **Servings:** 4
Ingredients:

- 2 cups mixed fresh fruit (such as berries, kiwi, pineapple, and grapes)
- 1 cup Greek yogurt
- 1 tablespoon honey
- 1/2 teaspoon vanilla extract
- 1/4 cup chopped nuts (such as almonds, walnuts, or pecans)

Instructions:

1. Wash and chop the fresh fruit into bite-sized pieces.
2. Mix the Greek yogurt, honey, and vanilla extract in a small bowl until well combined.
3. In a separate dry pan, toast the chopped nuts over medium heat for a few minutes until fragrant and lightly browned.
4. Toss the fresh fruit with the Greek yogurt mixture in a large mixing bowl until well coated.
5. Divide the fruit salad into 4 serving bowls or plates, and sprinkle with the toasted nuts.

Nutritional Values: Calories: 181 kcal Carbohydrates: 24 g Protein: 11 g Fat: 5 g Sodium: 48 mg Fiber: 3 g Sugar: 19 g

Frozen Yogurt Bark

Preparation time: 10 minutes Freezing time: 2-3 hours **Servings:** 6
Ingredients:

- 2 cups nonfat Greek yogurt
- 2 tablespoons honey
- 1/2 teaspoon vanilla extract
- 1/4 cup chopped mixed nuts (e.g., almonds, pistachios, walnuts)
- 1/4 cup mixed berries (e.g., strawberries, blueberries, raspberries)

Instructions:

1. Whisk together the Greek yogurt, honey, and vanilla extract in a medium mixing bowl until smooth.
2. Pour the mixture onto a baking sheet lined with parchment paper, spreading it into an even layer about 1/4 inch thick.
3. Sprinkle the chopped nuts and mixed berries over the top of the yogurt mixture, pressing them in gently.
4. Place the baking sheet in the freezer for 2-3 hours or until the yogurt has frozen solid.
5. Remove the baking sheet from the freezer and break the frozen yogurt bark into pieces.
6. Serve immediately or store in an airtight container in the freezer for up to 2 weeks.

Nutritional Values: Calories: 100 Fat: 3.5g Carbohydrates: 10g Fiber: 1g Protein: 8g Sodium: 25mg

Baked Apple with Cinnamon and Honey

Preparation time: 10 minutes **Cooking Time:** 25 minutes **Servings:** 4
Ingredients:

- 4 medium apples
- 2 tbsp. honey
- 1 tsp cinnamon
- 1/4 cup water
- Optional toppings: chopped nuts, Greek yogurt

Instructions:

1. Preheat the oven to 375°F (190°C).
2. Wash the apples and remove the core from the center of each apple, leaving the bottom intact.
3. Place the apples in a baking dish and drizzle them with honey.
4. Sprinkle cinnamon over the apples and pour water into the bottom of the dish.
5. Bake the apples for 20-25 minutes or until they are soft and tender.

6. Remove the apples from the oven and let them cool for a few minutes.

7. Serve warm baked apples with optional toppings such as chopped nuts or a dollop of Greek yogurt.

Nutritional Values: Calories: 105 kcal Fat: 0.3 g Carbohydrates: 28.1 g Fiber: 4.5 g Protein: 0.5 g Sodium: 1 mg

Homemade Banana Ice Cream

Preparation time: 10 minutes **Cooking Time:** 0 minutes Freezing time: 4-6 hours **Servings:** 4
Ingredients:

- 4 ripe bananas peeled and sliced.
- 1/4 cup unsweetened almond milk
- 1 tsp pure vanilla extract
- 1/4 tsp ground cinnamon
- 1/4 cup mixed nuts (such as almonds, cashews, and pistachios), chopped.

Instructions:

1. Place the sliced bananas on a baking sheet lined with parchment paper and freeze for at least 4 hours or until solid.

2. Once the bananas are frozen, add them to a food processor with almond milk, vanilla extract, and cinnamon. Process until the mixture is smooth and creamy, scraping down the sides of the food processor as needed.

3. Transfer the banana mixture to a freezer-safe container and fold in the chopped mixed nuts.

4. Freeze for 2-3 hours or until the ice cream is firm.

5. Let the ice cream sit at room temperature for 5-10 minutes before serving to soften slightly.

Nutritional Values: Calories: 138 Fat: 4.4g Saturated Fat: 0.6g Sodium: 1mg Carbohydrates: 25.3g Fiber: 3.4g Sugar: 13.9g Protein: 2.3g

Mixed Berry and Yogurt Parfait

Preparation time: 10 minutes. **Servings:** 2
Ingredients:

- 1 cup mixed berries (strawberries, blueberries, raspberries, blackberries)
- 1 cup plain Greek yogurt.
- 2 tablespoons honey

- 1/4 cup chopped walnuts.
- 1/4 teaspoon vanilla extract

Instructions:

1. Rinse the berries and pat them dry with a paper towel.

2. Mix the Greek yogurt, honey, chopped walnuts, and vanilla extract in a small bowl.

3. Layer the berries and the yogurt mixture in two small glasses or jars, alternating between the two.

4. Garnish the top with extra berries and a sprinkle of chopped walnuts.

5. Serve chilled.

Nutritional Values: Calories: 244 kcal Fat: 9.9 g Saturated Fat: 1.1 g Carbohydrates: 28.6 g Fiber: 3.9 g Protein: 15.2 g Sodium: 53 mg

Chia Seed Pudding with Mixed Fruit

Preparation time: 5 minutes Chilling time: 2-3 hours **Servings:** 4
Ingredients:

- 1 cup unsweetened almond milk
- 1/4 cup chia seeds
- 1-2 tablespoons honey
- 1 teaspoon vanilla extract
- 1 cup mixed fruit (such as berries, sliced banana, or diced mango)

Instructions:

1. Whisk together the almond milk, chia seeds, honey, and vanilla extract in a mixing bowl.

2. Let the mixture sit for a few minutes, then whisk again to prevent clumping.

3. Cover the bowl and refrigerate for at least 2-3 hours or overnight until the mixture thickens and the chia seeds soften.

4. Before serving, stir the pudding to ensure an even consistency.

5. Divide the pudding into 4 bowls or jars and top with mixed fruit.

6. Serve immediately or store in the refrigerator for up to 3 days.

Nutritional Values: Calories: 105 Fat: 5g Carbohydrates: 15g Fiber: 6g Protein: 3g Sodium: 59mg

Mixed Berry Crumble with Oatmeal Topping

Preparation time: 15 minutes **Cooking Time:** 40-45 minutes **Servings:** 6

Ingredients:

- 4 cups mixed berries (fresh or frozen)
- 2 tablespoons honey
- 1 tablespoon cornstarch
- 1/2 teaspoon cinnamon
- 1/4 teaspoon nutmeg
- 1/4 teaspoon salt
- 1 cup rolled oats.
- 1/4 cup whole wheat flour
- 1/4 cup chopped walnuts.
- 1/4 cup honey
- 1/4 cup unsweetened applesauce
- 2 tablespoons olive oil
- 1/2 teaspoon vanilla extract

Instructions:

1. Preheat oven to 350°F (175°C).
2. Toss the mixed berries, honey, cornstarch, cinnamon, nutmeg, and salt in a mixing bowl.
3. Pour the berry mixture into an 8x8-inch baking dish.
4. Combine the oats, whole wheat flour, chopped walnuts, honey, applesauce, olive oil, and vanilla extract in a separate mixing bowl.
5. Stir the oat mixture until it is evenly combined.
6. Sprinkle the oat mixture over the top of the berry mixture.
7. Bake the mixed berry crumble in the oven for 40-45 minutes, until the top is golden brown, and the filling is bubbling.
8. Allow the crumble to cool for 10-15 minutes before serving.

Nutritional Values: Calories: 250 kcal Protein: 4g Fat: 10g Carbohydrates: 40g Fiber: 5g Sodium: 110mg

Lemon and Blueberry Oatmeal Bars

Preparation time: 15 minutes **Cooking Time:**

30 minutes **Servings:** 12 bars

Ingredients:

- 1 1/2 cups rolled oats.
- 1/2 cup almond flour
- 1/4 cup honey
- 1/4 cup unsweetened applesauce
- 2 tbsp. coconut oil, melted.
- 1 tsp vanilla extract
- 1/2 tsp baking powder
- 1/4 tsp salt
- 1 lemon zested and juiced.
- 1 cup fresh blueberries

Instructions:

1. Preheat the oven to 350°F (175°C) and line an 8-inch square baking dish with parchment paper.
2. Combine the rolled oats, almond flour, baking powder, and salt in a large mixing bowl.
3. Whisk together the honey, applesauce, melted coconut oil, vanilla extract, lemon juice, and lemon zest in a separate bowl.
4. Pour the wet ingredients into the dry ingredients and stir until well combined.
5. Gently fold in the blueberries.
6. Transfer the mixture to the prepared baking dish and press firmly to make an even layer.
7. Bake for 25-30 minutes or until golden brown and set.
8. Let the oatmeal bars cool completely before slicing them into 12 bars.

Nutritional Values: Calories: 135 kcal Fat: 6.2 g Carbohydrates: 19.5 g Fiber: 2.1 g Protein: 2.5 g Sodium: 52 mg

Homemade Granola Bars

Preparation time: 20 minutes **Cooking Time:** 25 minutes **Servings:** 12 bars

Ingredients:

- 1 1/2 cups rolled oats.
- 1/2 cup almonds, chopped.
- 1/2 cup pecans, chopped.
- 1/2 cup dried cranberries
- 1/2 cup dried apricots, chopped.
- 1/4 cup honey

- 1/4 cup unsweetened applesauce
- 1/4 cup coconut oil
- 1 tsp vanilla extract
- 1/2 tsp ground cinnamon
- 1/4 tsp salt

Instructions:

1. Preheat oven to 350°F and line an 8-inch square baking dish with parchment paper.
2. Combine the oats, chopped nuts, dried cranberries, and chopped apricots in a large mixing bowl.
3. Whisk together the honey, applesauce, coconut oil, vanilla extract, ground cinnamon, and salt in a separate mixing bowl.
4. Pour the wet ingredients over the dry ingredients and mix until thoroughly combined.
5. Pour the mixture into the prepared baking dish and press firmly with a spatula to create an even layer.
6. Bake in the oven for 25 minutes or until the edges are golden brown.
7. Remove from the oven and allow to cool completely in the baking dish.
8. Once cooled, remove the granola mixture from the baking dish by pulling up the edges of the parchment paper.
9. Cut into 12 bars and store in an airtight container in the refrigerator.

Nutritional Values: Calories: 225 Fat: 13g Saturated Fat: 5g Cholesterol: 0mg Sodium: 55mg Carbohydrates: 25g Fiber: 4g Sugar: 13g Protein: 4g

Chocolate and Almond Butter

Preparation time: 15 minutes **Cooking Time:** 0 minutes **Servings:** 16
Ingredients:

- 1 cup rolled oats.
- 1/2 cup almond butter
- 1/4 cup honey
- 1/4 cup unsweetened cocoa powder
- 1/4 cup chocolate chips
- 1/4 cup chopped almonds.

- 1/4 cup ground flaxseed
- 1 teaspoon vanilla extract
- 1/4 teaspoon sea salt

Instructions:

1. Combine rolled oats, almond butter, honey, unsweetened cocoa powder, chocolate chips, chopped almonds, ground flaxseed, vanilla extract, and sea salt in a large mixing bowl. Stir well to combine.
2. Using a cookie scoop or tablespoon, roll the mixture into small balls and place them on a parchment-lined baking sheet.
3. Refrigerate for at least 1 hour to set.
4. Store the protein balls in an airtight container in the refrigerator for up to 1 week.

Nutritional Values: Calories: 128 Fat: 7.8g Saturated Fat: 1.5g Cholesterol: 0mg Carbohydrates: 13.3g Fiber: 2.5g Sugar: 6.8g Protein: 3.6g Sodium: 39mg

Fresh Fruit and Yogurt Smoothie

Preparation time: 5 minutes **Cooking Time:** 0 minutes **Servings:** 2
Ingredients:

- 1 cup plain Greek yogurt.
- 1 cup mixed fresh fruit (such as berries, mango, and banana)
- 1/2 cup unsweetened almond milk
- 1/2 teaspoon vanilla extract
- 1 tablespoon honey (optional)

Instructions:

1. In a blender, combine the Greek yogurt, mixed fruit, almond milk, vanilla extract, and honey (if using).
2. Blend until smooth and creamy.
3. Taste and adjust sweetness as needed by adding more honey, if desired.
4. Pour into glasses and serve immediately.

Nutritional Values: Calories: 146 kcal Fat: 4 g Carbohydrates: 19 g Fiber: 2 g Protein: 11 g Sodium: 51 mg Potassium: 301 mg

Greek Yogurt and Mixed Berry Popsicles

Preparation time: 10 minutes Freezing time: 4-6

hours **Servings:** 6
Ingredients:
- 1 cup Greek yogurt
- 1 cup mixed berries (fresh or frozen)
- 1 tbsp. honey
- 1/2 cup unsweetened almond milk
- 1 tsp vanilla extract

Instructions:
1. Combine Greek yogurt, mixed berries, honey, almond milk, and vanilla extract in a blender. Blend until smooth.
2. Pour the mixture into popsicle molds.
3. Freeze for 4-6 hours or until fully frozen.
4. To remove the popsicles from the molds, run them under warm water for a few seconds until they slide out easily.

Nutritional Values: Calories: 80 kcal Carbohydrates: 11g Protein: 5g Fat: 2g Fiber: 1g Sodium: 20mg

Blueberry and Lemon Yogurt Cake

Preparation time: 15 minutes **Cooking Time:** 45 minutes **Servings:** 12
Ingredients:
- 1 and 1/2 cups all-purpose flour
- 1/2 cup whole wheat flour
- 1/2 cup rolled oats.
- 1 teaspoon baking powder
- 1/2 teaspoon baking soda
- 1/4 teaspoon salt
- 1 cup plain Greek yogurt.
- 1/2 cup honey
- 1/3 cup vegetable oil
- 2 large eggs
- 1 teaspoon vanilla extract
- 2 tablespoons lemon zest
- 1 and 1/2 cups fresh or frozen blueberries

Instructions:
1. Preheat the oven to 350°F. Grease a 9-inch round cake pan and set aside.
2. Whisk together the all-purpose flour, whole wheat flour, rolled oats, baking powder, baking soda, and salt in a large mixing bowl.

3. In a separate mixing bowl, whisk together the Greek yogurt, honey, vegetable oil, eggs, vanilla extract, and lemon zest until well combined.
4. Pour the wet ingredients into the dry ingredients and stir until just combined.
5. Gently fold in the blueberries.
6. Pour the batter into the prepared cake pan and smooth the top with a spatula.
7. Bake for 40-45 minutes, or until a toothpick inserted into the center of the cake comes out clean.
8. Allow the cake to cool in the pan for 10 minutes, then remove it and transfer it to a wire rack to cool completely.
9. Slice and serve.

Nutritional Values: Calories: 214 Fat: 8g Saturated Fat: 1g Cholesterol: 31mg Sodium: 122mg
Carbohydrates: 32g Fiber: 2g Sugar: 15g Protein: 6g

Chocolate and Banana Oatmeal Cookies

Preparation time: 15 minutes **Cooking Time:** 15 minutes **Servings:** 12 cookies
Ingredients:
- 1 ripe banana, mashed.
- 1/4 cup unsweetened applesauce
- 1/4 cup honey
- 1/4 cup almond butter
- 1 tsp vanilla extract
- 1 1/2 cups rolled oats.
- 1/4 cup almond flour
- 1/4 cup cocoa powder
- 1/2 tsp baking powder
- 1/4 tsp salt
- 1/4 cup dark chocolate chips

Instructions:
1. Preheat the oven to 350°F (175°C) and line a baking sheet with parchment paper.
2. Whisk together the mashed banana, applesauce, honey, almond butter, and vanilla extract in a large bowl until smooth.

3. Combine the rolled oats, almond flour, cocoa powder, baking powder, and salt in another bowl.

4. Add the dry ingredients to the wet ingredients and stir until well combined.

5. Fold in the dark chocolate chips.

6. Use a cookie scoop or spoon to drop dough onto the prepared baking sheet, spacing them about 2 inches apart.

7. Bake for 12-15 minutes or until the cookies are set.

8. Allow the cookies to cool on the baking sheet for a few minutes before transferring them to a wire rack to cool completely.

Nutritional Values: Calories: 130 Fat: 5g Saturated Fat: 1g Cholesterol: 0mg Carbohydrates: 20g Fiber: 3g Sugar: 10g Protein: 3g Sodium: 60mg

Roasted Peaches with Greek Yogurt

Preparation time: 10 minutes **Cooking Time:** 20 minutes **Servings:** 4

Ingredients:

- 4 ripe peaches halved and pitted.
- 2 teaspoons olive oil
- 1 teaspoon cinnamon
- 1/4 teaspoon nutmeg
- 1/4 teaspoon ginger
- 1/4 teaspoon salt
- 1 cup nonfat Greek yogurt
- 2 tablespoons honey

Instructions:

1. Preheat the oven to 375°F (190°C).

2. Combine the olive oil, cinnamon, nutmeg, ginger, and salt in a small bowl.

3. Brush the cut sides of the peaches with the oil mixture.

4. Place the peaches cut side down on a baking sheet lined with parchment paper.

5. Roast the peaches in the oven for 15-20 minutes or until tender and caramelized.

6. While the peaches are roasting, mix the Greek yogurt and honey in a small bowl.

7. Serve the roasted peaches warm, topped with a dollop of the Greek yogurt and honey mixture.

Nutritional Values: Calories: 136 kcal Fat: 3 g Carbohydrates: 23 g Fiber: 2 g Protein: 8 g Sodium: 164 mg

Saturated Fat: 3 g Carbohydrates: 14 g Fiber: 3 g Sugar: 7 g Protein: 3 g Sodium: 60 mg

Meal Plan

DAY	BREAKFAST	LUNCH	DINNER	SNACK	DESSERTS
1	Greek Yogurt Parfait Berries and Granola	Lentil Soup with Whole	Quinoa Salad with Roasted Vegetables	Turkey and Avocado Lettuce Wraps	Baked Apple with Cinnamon and Honey
2	Berry and Spinach Smoothie Bowl	Grilled Salmon with Roasted Vegetable	Cobb Salad with Hard-Boiled Eggs	Greek Yogurt with Mixed Berries	Homemade Granola Bars
3	Broccoli And Feta Frittata	Chicken And Vegetable Stir-Fry	Sautéed Green Beans with Toasted Almonds	Roasted Vegetable and Hummus Wrap	Roasted Peaches With Greek Yogurt
4	Veggie Omelet with Spinach	Minestrone Soup with Whole-Grain Bread	Steamed Broccoli	Roasted Sweet Potato Wedges	Lemon And Blueberry Oatmeal Topping
5	Low Fat Breakfast Quesadilla	Grilled Chicken with Lemon and Herbs	Balsamic Roasted Carrots	Caprese salad	Chia Seed Pudding With Mixed Fruit
6	Steel-Cut Oatmeal whit Apples	Greek Lemon Chicken Soup	Garlic Roasted Cherry Tomatoes	Edamame With Sea Salt	Greek Yogurt and Mixed Berry Popsicles
7	Chia Seed Pudding with Apples	Grilled Chicken Caesar Salad	Grilled Eggplant With Balsamic Glaze	Carrots And Celery Sticks	Frozen Yogurt Bark
8	Chia Seed Pudding with Almond Milk	Turkey Meatloaf	Spicy Roasted	Spicy Roasted Cauliflower	Chocolate And Almond Butter
9	Baked Eggs With Cherry Tomatoes and Herbs	Chicken and Vegetable Lettuce Wraps	Roasted Butternut Squash with Maple Syrup	Trail Mix with Nuts	Mixed Berry and Yogurt Parfait
10	Smoked Salmon and Cucumber	Mediterranean Quinoa Salad	Sautéed Spinach With Garlic and Lemon	Roasted Chickpeas with Spices	Chocolate And Banana
11	Spinach and Mushroom Breakfast Skillet	Broccoli and Cheddar Soup	Lemon Garlic Pork Chops	Carrots and Celery Sticks	Homemade Granola Bars
12	Chia Seed Pudding with Almond Milk	Roasted Asparagus With Lemon and Garlic	Vegetable and Quinoa Soup	Trail Mix with Nuts	Chocolate and Banana Oatmeal Cookies
13	Whole-Grain Banana Pancakes	Grilled Chicken Breasts	Sautéed Spinach with Garlic and Lemon	Hummus With Whole-Grain Pita Chips	Chia Seed Pudding With Mixed Fruit
14	Cottage Cheese And Berry Breakfast Bowl	Spicy Shrimp and Vegetable Stir-fry	Grilled Salmon with Roasted Vegetable	Roasted Sweet Potatoes	Mixed Berry and Yogurt Parfait
15	Vegan Breakfast Tacos	Grilled Tuna Steak with Steamed Broccoli	Beef and vegetable Kebabs	Cottage Cheese With Mixed Berries	Chocolate And Almond Butter
16	Quinoa Breakfast Bowl	Seared Sea Scallops	Broccoli and Cheddar Soup	Roasted Nuts with Cinnamon and Honey	Fresh Fruit and Yogurt Smoothie
17	Greek Yogurt Parfait Berries and Granola	Spicy Roasted Cauliflower	Chicken And Vegetable Stir-Fry	Edamame with Sea Salt	Frozen Yogurt Bark
18	Avocado Toast with Poached Egg	Sautéed Spinach with Garlic and Lemon	Sweet Potato and Black Bean Soup	Quinoa and vegetable Stuffed Bell Peppers	Greek Yogurt and Mixed Berry Popsicles
19	Berry And Spinach Smoothie Bowl	Lemon and Herb Baked Salmon	Blackened Catfish with Collard Greens	Steamed or Roasted Broccoli	Homemade Granola Bars
20	Blueberry and Almond Butter Overnight Oats	Seared Sea Scallops	Steamed Broccoli	Roasted Vegetable and Hummus Wrap	Mixed Beery Crumble with Oatmeal Topping
21	Low-Fat Yogurt and Fruit Smoothies	Blackened Catfish with Collard Greens	Roasted Butternut Squash with Maple Syrup	Roasted Beets with Goat Cheese	Blueberry and Lemon Yogurt Cake

22	Peanut Butter and Banana Smoothie	Grilled Flank Steak with Roasted Vegetables	Grilled Asparagus with Lemon and Parmesan	Steamed Green Beans	Whole-Grain Apple Muffins
23	Smoked Salmon and Cucumber	Lemon Garlic Pork Chops	Sautéed Green Beans with Toasted Almonds	Carrot and Celery Sticks	Banana And Oatmeal
24	Cottage Cheese and Berry Breakfast Bowl	Greek Turkey Burgers	Quinoa Salad with Roasted Vegetables	Baked Sweet Potato Chips	Homemade Banana Ice
25	Avocado Toast with Poached Egg	Beef and vegetable Kebabs	Balsamic Roasted Carrots	Greek Yogurt with Mixed Berries	Mixed Berry and Yogurt
26	Veggie Omelet with Spinach	Baked Turkey Breast	Sautéed Spinach with Garlic and Lemon	Trail Mix with Nuts	Mixed Berry and Oatmeal
27	Whole-Grain Banana Pancakes	Grilled Chicken Caesar Salad	Roasted Asparagus With Lemon and Garlic	Greek Yogurt with Mixed Berries	Strawberry And Almond
28	Vegan Breakfast Tacos	Lemon and Herb Baked Salmon	Seared Sea Scallops	Baked Sweet Potato Chips	Grilled Pineapple
29	Low-Fat Yogurt and Fruit Smoothie	Turkey Meatloaf	Balsamic Roasted Carrots	Roasted Nuts with Cinnamon and Honey	Blueberry And Lemon
30	Whole-Grain Banana Pancakes	Sautéed Spinach with Garlic and Lemon	Chicken And Vegetable Stir-Fry	Whole-Grain Crackers with Low-Fat Cheese	Apple And Cinnamon

Conversion Table

Ingredient	Unit	Equivalent
Flour (all-purpose)	cups	1 cup = 120 grams
Flour (all-purpose)	ounces	1 ounce = 28 grams
Sugar (granulated)	cups	1 cup = 200 grams
Sugar (granulated)	ounces	1 ounce = 28 grams
Butter	cups	1 cup = 227 grams
Butter	tablespoons	1 tablespoon = 14 grams
Milk	cups	1 cup = 240 milliliters
Water	cups	1 cup = 240 milliliters
Honey	cups	1 cup = 340 grams
Honey	tablespoons	1 tablespoon = 21 grams
Yeast (instant)	teaspoons	1 teaspoon = 3 grams
Salt	teaspoons	1 teaspoon = 5 grams
Baking powder	teaspoons	1 teaspoon = 5 grams
Baking soda	teaspoons	1 teaspoon = 5 grams
Cocoa powder	tablespoons	1 tablespoon = 5 grams
Chocolate (chips or chunks)	cups	1 cup = 175 grams
Nuts (chopped)	cups	1 cup = 120 grams
Oats (rolled)	cups	1 cup = 90 grams
Oil (olive, vegetable, etc.)	tablespoons	1 tablespoon = 15 milliliters
Yogurt	cups	1 cup = 240 grams
Cream (heavy or whipping)	cups	1 cup = 240 milliliters
Cheese (grated)	cups	1 cup = 120 grams
Egg	large	1 large egg = approximately 50 grams
Vanilla extract	teaspoons	1 teaspoon = 5 milliliters

Mediterranean Diet
Cookbook
for
Beginners

1800 days of easy and
delicious recipes for eating healthy
and living well

GET YOUR BONUS NOW!

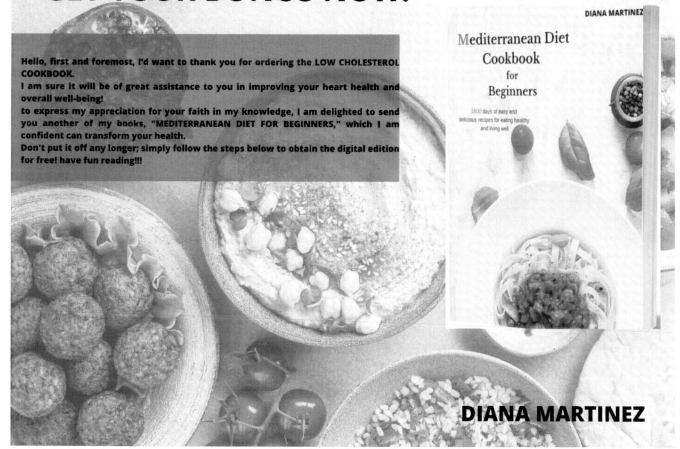

DIANA MARTINEZ

Mediterranean Diet
Cookbook
for
Beginners

1800 days of easy and
delicious recipes for eating healthy
and living well

DIANA MARTINEZ

Conclusion

As we come to the end of this book, I want to leave you with a message about the importance of following a meal plan that is both simple and sustainable. Getting caught up in the latest food trends or fad diets can be tempting, but a healthy and balanced diet doesn't have to be complicated or expensive.

By focusing on simple, readily available, affordable whole foods, you can create a meal plan that supports your health and respects your budget and time constraints. Eating well doesn't have to mean sacrificing flavor or enjoyment; countless delicious and nutritious recipes out there use essential ingredients and can be prepared quickly.

Most importantly, it's crucial to remember that our health is our most asset. By prioritizing our health and well-being through our food choices, we invest in ourselves, which will pay off in the long run. Eating a balanced diet and caring for our bodies give us the best chance to live a happy and fulfilling life.

Living a healthy, active, and balanced lifestyle is crucial for our well-being and happiness. Caring for our bodies and minds can increase our energy levels, reduce stress, and improve our overall quality of life.

One of the critical components of a healthy lifestyle is regular physical activity. Exercise has been shown to have numerous advantages, including reducing the risk of chronic diseases, improving mental health, and boosting cognitive function. Whether going for a walk, taking a yoga class, or hitting the gym, finding a form of physical activity you enjoy can make all the difference in your overall health and well-being.

But living a healthy lifestyle isn't just about exercise; it also involves making conscious choices about what we eat and drink. Eating a balanced diet with plenty of fruits, vegetables, whole grains, and lean proteins can provide our bodies with the nutrients and energy needed to thrive. On the other hand, consuming too many processed or sugary foods can lead to various health problems, including obesity, diabetes, and heart disease.

Another critical aspect of a healthy lifestyle is stress management. Chronic stress has been linked to various health problems, including depression, anxiety, and cardiovascular disease. Learning to manage stress through meditation, yoga, or deep breathing can help us feel more relaxed and at peace in our daily lives.

Finally, it's important to remember that a healthy lifestyle isn't just about the physical aspect; it also involves caring for our mental and emotional health. This can include engaging in activities that bring us joy and fulfillment, spending time with loved ones, and seeking professional help.

In conclusion, a healthy, active, and balanced lifestyle is essential for our overall well-being and happiness. By prioritizing physical activity, healthy eating, stress management, and mental and emotional health, we can live a life full of vitality and meaning. So, let's commit to ourselves to take care of our bodies and minds and live our best lives possible.

As we end this book, I want to express my sincere gratitude to you, the reader. Sharing my thoughts and ideas has been an honor and a privilege. This book has provided you with valuable insights and inspiration.

We all have the power to create a life full of joy, purpose, and fulfillment. By caring for our bodies and minds, pursuing our passions and dreams, and cultivating meaningful relationships, we can create a life worth living.

Of course, there will always be challenges and obstacles along the way. Still, we can overcome anything that comes our way with the right mindset and tools. So, whether you are just beginning your journey or are already well on your way, I encourage you to keep pushing forward, learning, and growing, and never giving up on your dreams.

As you progress from this book, I wish you all the best. May you find joy and fulfillment in everything you do, and may you never lose sight of the incredible potential within you. Remember that you can achieve great things and make a difference.

So, once again, thank you for taking the time to read this book, and I wish you all the best in your journey. May your life be filled with happiness, love, and all the blessings life offers.

Made in United States
North Haven, CT
14 September 2023

41465447R00067